"How we carry our bodies involves choice. *Back Trouble* clearly describes how to make choices that lead to balanced ease—a process that can help decrease many forms of back pain and increase overall well-being."

John H. M. Austin, M.D.
Radiologist
Columbia-Presbyterian Medical Center, NY

"The Alexander Technique has played an important and beneficient part in my life. I hope the clarity and simplicity of the Technique as laid out in Ms. Caplan's book will help to spread the general use of this most valuable tool."

John Houseman
Producer, Director, Actor

"Alexander students rid themselves of bad postural habits and not only appear to grow taller by two inches or so, they are helped to reach, with their bodies and their minds, an enviable degree of freedom of expression from which to embrace the rest of their training."

Michael Langham
Director, Theatre Center
The Juilliard School, NY

"I have found after working with you and using the Alexander method a terrific relief from the usual lower back pain I've had. Thanks, Debby."

Jim Dine
Artist

"Deborah Caplan's book, *Back Trouble*, is excellent, readable, and gives details of her treatment not available before."

Edwin S. Stempler, M.D., F.A.C.S.
Orthopedic surgeon
Palm Springs, CA

"I believe Deborah's book is the clearest presentation of Alexander's work yet written."

Judith Trobe, M.A., P.T.
Physical therapist, NY

BACK TROUBLE

A NEW APPROACH TO PREVENTION AND RECOVERY

by Deborah Caplan, M.A., P.T.

Photographs by the author
Anatomical drawings by Nancy Schadt
Human figure drawings by Kristin Johnson

TRIAD PUBLISHING COMPANY   GAINESVILLE, FLORIDA

Printed in the United States of America

Published and distributed by
Triad Publishing Company, Inc.
1110 Northwest Eighth Avenue
Gainesville, Florida 32601

Library of Congress Cataloging-in-Publication Data

Caplan, Deborah, 1931-
Back trouble.

    Includes index.
    1. Backache -- popular words.   2. Backache -- prevention.
I. Title. (DNLM: 1. Backache -- prevention & control --
popular works.   WE 720 C244b)
RD768.C37   1987   617'.56   87-5851
ISBN 0-937404-26-8 (pbk.)

The exercises and other information in this book are not intended to substitute for medical diagnosis and treatment. Because each person and situation is unique, the author and publisher urge the reader to check with a qualified health professional before using a new health or exercise procedure.

To my mother, Alma Frank, in memory and gratitude

To Aaron and Leah

And to Larry

Contents

Foreword

BACK TROUBLE IS a frustrating problem for both patient and physician. Physicians are trained to relate signs and symptoms to specific diseases and to diagnose and treat accordingly. But, in the case of chronic back pain, it is often impossible to make a specific diagnosis, and most treatments fail. The patient, increasingly dependent on analgesics, gets frustrated and depressed, and the physician loses tolerance for the patient he cannot treat. As a result, more than ninety percent of patients in chronic pain clinics are there because of back pain.

The impact of back pain is felt not only by physician and patient, but by society as a whole. The costs of medical care and of absenteeism from the workplace amount to many billions each year—yes, billions. Back pain is the most expensive disease of the middle-aged worker.

What is even more alarming is that the number of people who have back trouble is increasing while our understanding of the condition remains inadequate and our treatment haphazard.

Can the situation be changed? And how?

Let me start by saying that little will change until the medical community becomes more open-minded about legitimate alternatives to conventional—but usually unsuccessful—medical therapies. The Alexander Technique is one such alternative. It is a system for teaching people how to best use their bodies in ordinary action to avoid or reduce unnecessary stress and pain. It is a system of postural education, a way of heightening the kinesthetic sense.

My own exposure to the Alexander Technique came about quite by accident. As the neurosurgical director of a busy spinal surgery service, I am constantly alert to the need for qualified physical therapists who are knowledgeable about spinal mechanics and, equally important, are interested in care of patients with either acute or chronic back ailments. Finding such therapists is difficult, and when one opened her office near the Westchester Medical Center, I was delighted.

What amazed me about this new therapist was that her office contained only a chair and a table with a mat, and yet the patients I sent to her were getting better faster. I soon discovered that she was teaching them how to use their bodies with the ease of movement for which the body was designed and intended. Oh, yes, she gave them specific exercises, but most importantly, she used the Alexander Technique.

Well, up until that point, the only Alexanders I had been familiar with were Alexander the Great and Alexander's Ragtime Band. F. M. Alexander was a new acquaintance. It is not my objective to tell you about him or the Technique since you have bought this exciting book. I will say, however, that the uniqueness of the Alexander approach is that it emphasizes using the mind and body in unity. This is undoubtedly the best way to care for the back and alleviate back pain.

The Alexander Technique stresses unification in an era of greater and greater medical subspecialization. It enables patients with back trouble to get better faster and stay better longer.

JACK STERN, M.D., PH.D.
Neurosurgical Director
Section of Spinal Surgery
Westchester Medical Center
New York Medical College
Valhalla, New York

Preface

I WAS TEN years old when I first met F. M. Alexander, and to this day what comes to mind when I think of him is his twinkling eyes, the elegant spats he loved to wear, and his nightly readings to us children from *Winnie the Pooh* and *The Wind in the Willows*. These memories date back to 1941, when Alexander spent time in the United States. During his stay here he established a small live-in school in Massachusetts, which I attended. At the school we received our usual academic instructions plus daily lessons from Alexander.

I again took lessons from Alexander after I graduated from college, this time traveling to England to do so. My appreciation of his work was naturally on a more adult level this time around. I have personally benefited from having the Alexander Technique as part of my daily life, and I have helped my patients derive similar benefits by integrating the technique into their physical therapy treatment.

I now want you to start applying Alexander's technique to your own daily activities. As a way to begin, I would like you to read an excerpt from Alexander's book, *The Use of the Self*, which is about good health and how we use our bodies:

". . . the most valuable knowledge we can possess is that of the use and functioning of the self, and of the means whereby the human individual may progressively raise the standard of his health and general well-being."

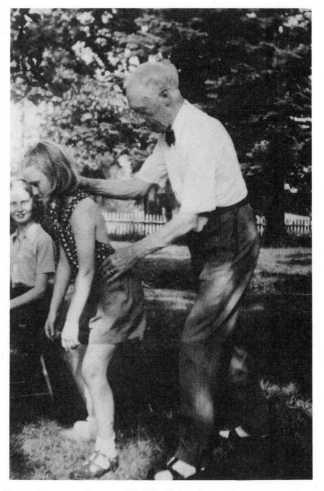

The author, age ten, and F. M. Alexander. *(Photo by Alma Frank)*

Acknowledgments

FIRST AND FOREMOST I want to express my deepest gratitude to Judith Trobe, physical therapist and teacher of the Alexander Technique, who provided many of the essential ingredients required for the completion of this book. Her constant support and assistance were invaluable to me. When the manuscript was ready to be critiqued by a physical therapy colleague, Judy took on the job. She devoted countless hours and meticulous care to this vital task, giving generously of her considerable knowledge and experience. The book is much enriched by her many contributions.

Without the assistance of my Alexander colleagues, this book could not have been written. I am most grateful for their recommendations and criticisms, and for the generosity of those who gave their time and Alexander skills by demonstrating for the instructive photographs. I want to thank Pamela Anderson, Pearl Ausubel, Ron Dennis, Joanne Howell, Carolyn Kitahata, Jane Kosminsky, Judith Leibowitz, Julia MacKenzie, Carolyn Monka, Ruth Belding Nardini, Thomas M. Nardini, Maria Parker, Eleanor Rosenthal, Mollie Schnoll, Jessica Wolf, and Andrew Zavada.

Early on in my writing efforts, I benefited from the instruction of a truly great teacher, Erika Duncan. She taught me to hear and trust my inner voice.

I would like to thank Ruth Randall who contributed greatly to making this book a reality by being so generous with her expertise.

I am indebted to John H. M. Austin, M.D. and Jack Stern, M.D. for their careful reading of the manuscript and many valuable recommendations.

I am most grateful for the expert assistance I received from Marcia Amsterdam, William P. Burks, M.D., Ralph Caplan, Laura Ferguson, Jean Frank, John Goldsmith, Henry Grossman, Dorothea von Haeften, Lenore Hecht, Arthur Lavine, Michael G. Neuwirth, M.D., Judith Rosen, Edwin S. Stempler, M.D., and Donna Zalichin.

It was a pleasure working with Nancy Schadt, who did the anatomical illustrations, and with Kristin Johnson, who did the human figure drawings. Thank you both.

Karen Tweedy-Holmes generously wrought her artistic magic and skill to give me beautiful prints of the instructive photographs.

I want to thank my editor, Rebecca Howard, and my publisher, Lorna Rubin, for their skilled assistance.

My Alexander students and patients inspired me to write this book and contributed greatly to my appreciation and understanding of Alexander's work.

My children, Aaron and Leah, never stopped supporting my writing efforts and tolerated my mood swings with great under- standing.

And finally, my boundless and undying gratitude to Larry King, who freely gave of his much needed support and many talents throughout the entire project.

BACK TROUBLE

Introduction

"The Next Best Thing To a Magic Wand"

"Can you cure my back pain?"

DOCTORS AND PHYSICAL THERAPISTS hear this question all the time. I have learned over many years with many patients that the variables affecting the human back are too numerous and too individual to permit a true cure, short of having a magic wand at one's disposal.

Undoubtedly you, too, have already learned that there is no magic treatment for back trouble, and you may feel victimized by your condition. There *is* a solution, however: you can learn to *use your back* in a way that will be immediately beneficial. All the heat, massage, traction, bed rest, spinal mobilization, exercises, acupuncture, medication, or surgery in the world will not undo the harmful effects of continual incorrect use of the back. Treatment is helpful, but its effects are often short-lived because every time you sit, stand, or bend incorrectly you risk re-injuring your back and preventing it from healing.

I think I have given my patients something almost as good as magic. I have taught them what to do and not do when their backs give them trouble, and how to reduce the frequency and duration of their episodes of pain. As a result, they no longer have to feel afraid and helpless when back pain does occur. Many consider themselves cured because they have been able to return to an active, essentially normal life-style.

Back Trouble: A New Approach to Prevention and Recovery contains the same kind of information and help. It gives step-by-step, clearly illustrated instructions on how you can take an active part in your own recovery.

Back Trouble teaches you to use your back in a way that heals. Learning how to use your back correctly will not only enable you to get better, it will help prevent further injury. I think you will find the process enjoyable as well as therapeutic. In sports and in your daily activities, you will move, work, and play with greater ease and less tension and fatigue.

Many of the instructions are based on the principles of the Alexander Technique, a logical, commonsense approach that teaches a way of using the body with less tension and more efficiency as you carry out your daily activities. Developed over a half-century ago by F. M. Alexander, this system of psycho-physical education has helped countless people with many different forms of tension and back pain. Although exploring the technique in its entirety requires the hands-on guidance of a teacher, many valuable Alexander principles can be conveyed, as I will do here, in words and illustrations.

An important theme of the Alexander Technique and of this book is that the *entire* spine and back must be used correctly if a painful condition in one area is to get better. Consequently, you will learn not only how to deal with lower back pain, but also neck, shoulder, and upper back problems.

The book begins with an explanation of why postural habits affect such problems as low back pain, neck pain, and arthritis.

This is followed by Alexander's own story and the ways his work is particularly helpful for those with back pain. It then describes the "Concepts of Good Use," an important part of the Alexander Technique.

The next three chapters focus on those parts of the body most relevant to spine and back problems. Each begins with a brief anatomy lesson to help you understand why certain ways of moving are harmful and others beneficial, and concludes with how correct use of the body can help specific medical problems.

Chapters 1 through 6 lay the foundation for the rest of the book and follow the same sequence of instruction I use with all my patients, whether they have problems in the neck, shoulders and upper back, or lower back. If you read them in sequence it will be easier to apply a new way of moving to your body.

As you work with this book you will learn important facts about using your back in a beneficial way, and you will gain the skills necessary to help you get better. You will come to realize, as I have during my many years of treating back problems, that "good use" of the back is essential for effective recovery. Using your back correctly is indeed powerful medicine for an ailing back.

1

Your Back Pain and How You Use Your Back

Disc trouble
Sciatica
Low back pain
Whiplash injury
Shoulder-arm pain
Neck pain
Pinched nerves
Arthritis in the spine
Round shoulders
Swayback

THERE IS A WAY TO MOVE that is beneficial to the body, and a way that is harmful; a way to move that increases the injured body's ability to heal itself, and another that interferes with this ability.

Look at the conditions listed above. Though they have varying causes and symptoms, they all have one thing in common: each can be made better or worse by the way you align and balance your head, neck, and back as you go about your daily activities.

Poor postural habits, such as sitting slumped or standing with an arched back, take the body out of good alignment and compress joint surfaces so tightly together that their movement is unnecessarily restricted. Your skeleton should be used in a way that allows its many joints to move freely. Your muscles, which support your skeleton and enable it to move around, frequently work too hard, or some muscles are overworked while others do not work enough. Ideally, all your muscles should work together in an efficient, balanced way.

GOOD "USE" VERSUS GOOD POSTURE

As you read this book, it may seem as though I am talking about the importance of having good, rather than bad, posture. In a limited sense I am, in that poor posture can interfere with the healing of a back problem and good posture in its true sense can hasten healing. However, using the word posture in this way is treading on dangerous ground because few people have an accurate understanding of what "good" posture is. When I asked a friend what came to mind when he thought of good posture, he said, "drill sergeants, parental admonitions, and strict school teachers." Another came up with "sitting up stiff and straight while my neck and back muscles get painfully tense." Most people think of good posture as uncomfortable and unattainable.

I object to the term, not only because of its "uncomfortable" connotation, but because it commits a serious sin of omission: it excludes consideration of what happens to the body in motion. Therefore, instead of talking about your posture, I will be referring to your *postural habits*, or to your *use*, or to your *habits of use*. These three terms are interchangeable and motion-oriented. They represent all the factors that determine how you use your body, whether beneficial or harmful, whether you are moving or at rest.

I will be teaching you some specifics of good and bad use so that you can detect and eliminate those aspects of your own habits of use that are harmful and contribute to your back pain. As you understand more about what good use entails, you will find that, merely by thinking about them, your postural habits start to improve.

THE IMPORTANCE OF GOOD USE

The human body has a remarkable capacity to repair itself, and postural habits that align the skeleton efficiently and enable the muscles to be used in a balanced way increase your body's ability to heal a back problem. Good use is also the most effective way of preventing a recurrence of back problems. Poor use, on the other hand, can actually prevent your back from getting better.

Suppose you have suffered a whiplash injury to your neck. The amount of tension you habitually have in your neck muscles and how you align your head and neck while walking, bending, or even talking on the phone will significantly affect how well and quickly you heal.

Or, you may have hurt your lower back by picking up a heavy object incorrectly. Your doctor has determined that you have injured a spinal disc, which is pressing on the sciatic nerve giving you pain down one leg. Your injury is to the structures of the spine. Therefore, how you align and muscularly support these structures will either help or hinder your recovery.

Perhaps you suffer from recurring back pain but do not know what brings it on. Years of poor postural habits are the likely cause. They should be replaced by beneficial ones.

Arthritis is a condition that affects the joints in the body, and joints have muscles crossing over them. Continually holding the muscles tight increases mechanical stress on the joints, so that moving becomes harder and more painful. Improved postural habits cannot make arthritis go away, but they can decrease your discomfort and help you keep your joints moving.

If you have had spinal surgery for a disc problem, you can help prevent a recurrence of problems above or below the site of the surgery by learning to use your abdominal and back muscles for support. Your abdominal muscles form part of a natural corset, and you need to learn how to use them effectively.

If you have experienced an episode of back pain, you may be afraid to move for fear of re-injuring yourself. Unfortunately, the very attempt to protect your body by being less active can make joints stiff and muscles weak.

Pinched nerves in the neck or lower back can occur when your spine is continually compressed by faulty postural habits. Constant spinal compression leaves less space for the nerve roots and may cause calcium deposits (osteophytes) to form, which can irritate the nerves. By learning to use your muscles to align your spine correctly, you can give the nerve roots more space and help prevent the formation of calcium deposits. Your first practical lesson in this book will teach you to reduce spinal compression so you will not continually hurt yourself.

Some of the conditions mentioned above, such as chronic low back pain, are most likely caused by poor habits of use, while others, such as neck pain resulting from a whiplash injury, are not. For all of them, however, the quality of your daily postural habits plays an important part in recovery.

Whether you are eighteen or eighty, learning to move in a way that is beneficial to your back is both necessary and effective. Everyone, regardless of age, can and should learn to move with maximum ease and improved alignment. Using your body then becomes a pleasurable as well as a healing experience.

THE MIND-BODY CONNECTION

Healing as a human endeavor has taken many forms throughout history, ranging from religious ritual to scientific exploration. Today, a new frontier in medical treatment is exploring how the conscious mind can influence the body to restore health.

Research has shown that people can be taught to change, at will, their heart rate, blood pressure, skin temperature, and brain waves. Studies using electromyography, a procedure that registers nerve-muscle activity, have demonstrated that people can attain more precise conscious control over their skeletal muscles than was previously thought possible.

It has long been recognized that some of the interaction between mind and body can be detrimental, causing conditions such as ulcers, high blood pressure, and tension headaches. We are now learning that conscious awareness and control of the body can be used to *restore* and *maintain* health.

A pioneer in this new field was a young actor named F. M. Alexander, who, at the turn of the century, was waging a personal battle for health. As he learned how much control he could have over his body by using conscious awareness, he began developing a process that enabled him to improve his total musculoskeletal functioning. This process has come to be known as the Alexander Technique.

As medicine moves further in the direction of health maintenance and explores ways in which patients can learn to help themselves, the Alexander Technique is becoming widely recognized for its therapeutic value.

2
Understanding the Alexander Technique

The best way of introducing you to this wonderful technique is with Alexander's own story.

FREDERICK MATTHIAS ALEXANDER was born in Australia in 1869. As a young man he became an actor, specializing in Shakespearean monologues. He was in his early twenties and already launched on a promising career when he began to be troubled by hoarseness while performing. The doctor he consulted told him that the mucous membranes of his throat were irritated and his vocal cords were inflamed. The medications prescribed by the doctor, as well as various other solutions suggested by his voice coaches, provided only temporary relief.

In his book *The Use of the Self*, in which he describes how he developed his technique, Alexander tells of his dilemma:

> The treatment I was receiving became less and less effective as time went on, and the trouble gradually increased until, after a few years, I found to my dismay that I had developed a condition of hoarseness which from time to time culminated in a complete loss of voice.

When Alexander lost his voice completely during a performance and the doctor had no better suggestion than to continue the ineffective treatments, Alexander asked him:

> "Is it not fair, then, to conclude that it was *something I was doing that evening in using my voice that was the cause of the trouble?*"

The doctor thought a moment and said, Yes, that must be so."

> "Can you tell me, then, *what it was that I did* that caused the trouble?"

The doctor admitted that he could not.

To find out what he was doing with his vocal mechanism while performing, Alexander set up mirrors so he could observe himself while reciting.

> I was particulary struck by three things that I saw myself doing. I saw that as soon as I started to recite, I tended to pull back the head, depress the larynx, and suck in breath through the mouth in such a way as to produce a gasping sound.

As Alexander became more skilled at self-observation, he discovered that he did the same thing during ordinary speaking, though to a lesser degree. And as his meticulous self-observation continued, he made further discoveries: first, when he used his head incorrectly by pulling it "back and down" (as he described it), his torso decreased in overall length and width because he arched his back and thrust his chest forward; and second, that he had unnecessary tension in his legs and arms.

He realized that he was dealing with a *total pattern* of misuse that involved his entire body, not just one small area! Alexander had made the important discovery that the way he *used* his body affected the way it *functioned* and, further, that the way he *used his entire body* affected the way *any one area of it functioned.*

He now knew that he needed to correct his total "habitual use" to cure his vocal difficulties.

Since Alexander's harmful use involved his entire body, he had to find out where to begin focusing his corrective efforts — with his faulty breathing, on his misuse of his larynx, or on his misuse of his head and torso. As he put it, "I found myself in a maze."

After many years of tireless investigation, Alexander finally discovered that his total pattern of misuse was initiated from the head down and involved his head, neck, and torso. That discovery led him to develop the basic characteristics of his technique:

The importance of the head-neck-torso unit.

The use of mental instructions to guide the body.

Inhibition as an important first step.

THE HEAD-NECK-TORSO UNIT

By correcting the way he used his head, neck, and torso, Alexander's other faulty habits (gasping in air, depressing his larynx, tensing his arms and legs) were instantly reduced, and they eventually disappeared. He was so struck by what happened that he wanted to find out whether this same kind of cause-and-effect applied to others as well. He began working with several people to get an answer and found that correcting their head-neck-torso integration did indeed enable them to get rid of many tension-related body problems and to carry out their daily activities with greater ease and efficiency.

MENTAL INSTRUCTIONS

To correct the misuse of his head, neck and torso, Alexander developed specific mental instructions to guide his body, which I call the *Concepts of Good Use* (he referred to them as "directions" or "orders"). He realized that using mental instructions to correct his harmful use was more trustworthy than relying on body feelings. After all, his faulty habits felt "right" by virtue of their long familiarity, whereas the improved use felt "wrong" because of its unfamiliarity.

"Obviously," Alexander stated, "any new use must feel different from the old, and if the old use felt right, the new use was bound to feel wrong." He described this inaccurate feedback from the body as "debauched kinesthesia" and said that "if it is possible for feeling to become untrustworthy as a means of direction, it should also be possible to make it trustworthy again." This, of course, is true: the kinesthetic, or body, sense, *does* become reliable as improved use is practiced for long periods of time.

INHIBITION

Surprisingly, Alexander's most challenging obstacle to solving his voice problem came *after* he had worked out the mental instructions (Concepts of Good Use). He found that no matter how long he repeated them to himself before reciting, their good effect on his body stopped, and his old faulty habits returned, as soon as he started to recite.

Again by repeated trial and error, Alexander discovered the reason for this failure. Since his habitual use (the one that had caused him his problem in the first place) was so closely associated with the act of reciting, it recurred *the instant he made the decision to recite.*

Alexander eventually overcame this obstacle by realizing he had omitted an important first step. He first had to make the conscious decision *not* to react in his familiar way to the idea of reciting. In other words, he had to say no to his habitual response before a new response could take its place. He used the word *inhibition* to refer to the conscious stopping of an habitual response.

"The immediate result of Alexandrian inhibition," according to Frank Pierce Jones, Ph.D., in his book, *Body Awareness in Action: A Study of the Alexander Technique*," is a sense of freedom, as if a heavy garment that had been hampering all of your movements has been removed."

In *The Use of the Self,* Alexander states that through repeatedly employing inhibition and conscious direction (the Concepts of Good Use), he eventually reached the point where the improved use automatically accompanied the decision to recite. He had found the solution to his voice difficulties.

In making these discoveries, Alexander learned a specific procedure for bringing his many harmful habits of use—of which he was formerly unaware—to the conscious level so that he could change them for the better. The procedure involved using not just his mind and not just his body, but a harmonious interaction between the two.

As Alexander's career in Australia gradually changed from acting to teaching "the work" (as he called it), he gained the attention and admiration of the medical profession. With the encouragement of physicians and friends, he went to England in 1904 to make his work better known. He taught successfully in London, attracting the attention of many in both the performing arts and the medical world.

In the early 1930s Alexander started his first program to train others to teach his technique. People came from all over the world to study with him and opened centers in their own countries to give lessons and train future teachers. Alexander was still teaching in London when he died in 1955, at the age of eighty-six.

THE ALEXANDER TECHNIQUE AND BACK PAIN

Although the benefits of Alexander's work are manifold, three aspects of his technique are particularly valuable for those with back pain.

Using the Whole Back Correctly

Alexander's approach—*dealing with the totality to solve a specific problem*—is particularly valuable when treating back pain. A problem may occur in one area of the back, but this area cannot heal unless the entire back is used in a well-integrated way.

Dealing with Gravity

Most people consider gravity to be a harmful, but unavoidable, burden our backs must bear. The fault, however, lies not with gravity or our uprightness, but with an inadequate use of one of our most important evolutionary gifts: *the ability to be aware of, and therefore control, our supporting musculature*. The Alexander Technique teaches us how to use this awareness and control to stop gravity from harming the back and let it begin actually helping. The ability to make this change is valuable for everyone. For those with back pain it is a necessity.

Eliminating Tension

Learning to do *less* with the body is one of the most useful aspects of Alexander's work for back pain sufferers. Doing less does not mean being less active, but rather, eliminating all the unnecessary muscle tension and harmful postural habits that can cause, and prolong, back pain.

As you begin learning to eliminate unnecessary muscle tension, you will be able to stop the tension cycle that invariably accompanies back problems. This cycle occurs because pain causes more tension, which in turn causes more pain, and so on. Many of my patients have found that by using the Alexander Technique they are able to stop this painful cycle themselves and thus avoid taking muscle relaxants and painkillers. They also feel more energetic, since they are not using so much of their energy in the form of unnecessary muscle tension.

3

The Four Concepts of Good Use

---

*"You can actually feel the difference in my body
when I 'think' to it?" asks the student.
"Yes, definitely," replies the Alexander teacher.*

EVEN THOUGH THE RESULT of an Alexander lesson is an efficient, easeful use of the body, the procedure the student goes through is primarily mental rather than physical.

Perhaps you have already attempted to improve your postural habits by making an heroic muscular effort to straighten your spine and pull your shoulders back. If so, you most likely discovered that the main result of your efforts was uncomfortable muscle tension.

This method did not work for Alexander, either. Instead, he found a way to consciously guide his body out of its accustomed postural habits and into a new, improved use. For guidelines he developed four specific Concepts of Good Use, which are mental instructions for different parts of the body. The first two Concepts deal with the head, neck, and torso. The second two are for the legs and shoulders.

Individuals who start to apply these Concepts to themselves will find their neck and shoulder muscles becoming less tense, their backs becoming longer, and their hip joints becoming freer. When Alexander teachers place their hands gently on a student's neck or back muscles during a lesson, they can feel these changes taking place.

You may wonder at first whether "thinking" to your body can actually change the amount of tension in your muscles. Let me assure you, as I do my patients, that it can. Changes in nerve and muscle activity produced just by thinking can be detected by electromyographic (EMG) equipment.

Studies using the Alexander Technique in conjunction with electromyography are described by F. P. Jones in his book, *Body Awareness in Action: A Study of the Alexander Technique.* In his experiments, Dr. Jones directed subjects to sit in their habitual relaxed position. Then he asked them, first, to "sit up straight" by their usual method and second, to achieve an improved sitting alignment by using the Alexander Technique. After the first instruction, subjects showed a marked increase in neck muscle tension on the EMG equipment, whereas after the second they had a decrease in tension and at the same time, a greater lengthening of the spine.

These are the Concepts of Good Use, which form an important part of the Alexander Technique:

    I.   *Allow your neck to release so that your head can balance forward and up.*
   II. *Allow your torso to release into length and width.*
  III. *Allow your legs to release away from your pelvis.*
  IV. *Allow your shoulders to release out to the sides.*

The four Concepts have an important characteristic in common: they all instruct you to *release* your muscles. Therefore, before explaining the Concepts, I want to clarify this term.

RELEASING YOUR MUSCLES

Unnecessary tension in the skeletal muscles is a major cause of back pain and can set the stage for injury to other structures of the back, such as the ligaments and joints. Tense muscles eventually become painful, lose their flexibility, and are more vulnerable to injury. So please do not impose more tension on your already hurting muscles by holding your shoulders back or walking around with your buttocks tight. You will learn to correct your harmful postural habits by releasing, not tensing, your muscles.

What Are Released Muscles?

Released muscles are those that are working *only as much as they need to, to perform a particular task.* Tense muscles, on the other hand, are doing more work than is necessary. Released muscles work efficiently; tense muscles work inefficiently.

How Will You Know When Your Muscles Are Released?

Your first attempts to consciously release your muscles may leave you confused and prompt you to ask yourself, "Am I doing it right?" or "Am I there yet?"

The answer to these questions will come from the way your muscles feel. Let me show you what I mean with the muscles in your hand. Make a fist with one hand, tensing the muscles in your wrist and fingers as much as possible. If you maintain this tension long enough, your hand will get tired and may even start to hurt. Now slowly let go of most of the tension, so you have a looser fist, and notice the change in the way your hand feels. The tiredness and discomfort will disappear.

It is possible to increase or decrease tension in this same way in your large postural muscles, even though the contrast in feeling will be harder to detect than it was in your hand.

My new patients describe having lessened sensation in the muscle groups they habitually hold tense except, unfortunately, for feelings of discomfort or pain. They have walked around with tense postural muscles, and yet they are unaware of doing so until pain develops. However, as they start to practice releasing, their ability to sense the state of their muscles increases.

Since the ability to release your muscles is a skill, the more you practice, the more ability and confidence you will gain. Even a momentary releasing of muscles usually held tight will benefit your body and begin training your muscles to work without unnecessary tension. Please do not think in terms of being "right" or "wrong" as you practice releasing, but rather of gradually developing an important skill involving both your mind and body.

Some Ways To Practice Releasing Muscles

You may feel, as many do, that releasing your muscles is beyond your conscious ability. Let me show you that you can, indeed, learn this skill.

Here is a simple releasing exercise you can do while you continue reading. Pick up a cup as though you were going to drink from it (you can pretend to be holding a cup if you do not have one handy). Hold the cup close to your mouth and release as much tension from your neck, shoulder, and raised arm as you can without moving the cup. What did you feel? Did you feel a lessening of tension? If so, the amount of tension you just gave up was all unnecessary tension.

What you just accomplished was *releasing* your muscles. You did not relax them because they were still working to hold your arm up (muscles are *relaxed* only when they are not doing any work at all). Repeat the exercise, this time paying particular attention to the change in feeling in your neck and shoulder muscles as you get rid of the unnecessary muscle tension.

The next releasing exercise is for the parts of your body that may become tense when you work at a desk. Sit at a desk or table and start writing something that requires very little concentration, such as the months of the year or your address. As you write, think of releasing the tension in your neck and shoulders. As the releasing occurs, your shoulders may lower slightly and feel freer and less tired. Notice how you are holding your pen: are you using more tension than you need? You will probably find that you can write just as efficiently with less grip in your fingers, wrist, and arm. Notice how your handwriting changes as the tension in your arm and hand lessens. Now, still writing, be aware of any unnecessary tension you may have in your legs and feet. Are you holding your knees tightly together? Are you tensing your ankles and feet? If so, consciously release this tension the same way you released the tension in your hand after you made a fist. The best position for your feet is on the floor, either comfortably apart or with ankles crossed.

The unnecessary tension you released throughout your body while writing may return as soon as you think of something else. Do not be discouraged; simply undo the tension each time you become aware of it. Gradually your body will learn to stay in a more tension-free state as you write.

You may find it helpful to think of muscle tension as "muscle noise" and of your muscles becoming "quiet" as you release them. This analogy is not just a fanciful one. Electromyographic equipment includes a speaker to convert the electrical activity of muscles into sound (the sound produced is similar to that of static on a radio). As you decrease your muscle tension, think of this muscle noise decreasing so that your body becomes more quiet.

You can also have a friend help you practice releasing. Sit in a straight chair with your hips all the way back in the seat so you can lean against the back of the chair without slumping. Have your friend very gently turn your head from side to side. Does your head turn easily or does it feel (to your friend) like it is stuck in one position? Now think of your neck muscles releasing. You will discover that as you think of releasing, your head will be easier to turn.

Check the releasing in your legs by putting one hand on top of each thigh and gently shaking your thigh muscles from side to side with quick hand motions. The freer your leg muscles are, the more they will respond to being shaken.

CONCEPTS I AND II

The first two Concepts of Good Use are interdependent and their purpose is to bring about an integrated, beneficial use of the head, neck, and torso. An important effect of these two Concepts is that they encourage you to maintain length in your spine. The spine is a curved, flexible structure. It can either be posturally compressed, which is harmful, or posturally lengthened, which is beneficial.

Concept I: Allow Your Neck To Release
So Your Head Can Balance Forward and Up

The well-being of the spine depends upon head balance. When your neck muscles are held tight, your head presses down on your neck and compresses your entire spine. Therefore, you have to first eliminate this incorrect use of your head (Concept I) before your spine can lengthen (Concept II).

Give yourself the instruction to *release your neck muscles so your head can balance forward and up* off your neck instead of being pulled back and down. The forward instruction does not mean that your head moves forward of the rest of your body in space; it is telling you to undo a backward pull on your head. Alexander's use of the word "up" always means away from the top of the spine (this will, of course, not be toward the ceiling if you are lying down or bending over), and the purpose of the up concept is to eliminate any muscle tension that pulls the head down onto the neck. Head "forward and up" is something you allow to happen by releasing your neck muscles. It will enable your head to be poised freely on top of your neck.

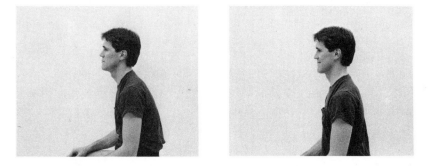

(Left) **Incorrect: Head pulled back and down.** *(Right)* **Correct: Head releasing forward and up.**

To feel the difference between head "back and down" and "forward and up" on yourself, place one hand gently around the back of your neck with your little finger under your head. Now tighten the muscles under your hand. Your hand will feel how the curve in your neck changes and the back of your head comes closer to the bottom of your neck. This is head "back and down." To change it to "forward and up," release the tension in your neck muscles so that your head can rotate forward. Even though your face lowers slightly, the overall effect is that your entire head will ease up off your neck, and the back of your neck will become longer because it is not compressed.

Concept II: Allow Your Torso To Release into Length and Width

When I ask you to apply the concept of *length* to your torso, I am not referring to some magical activity your body cannot perform, but rather to one of the many postural choices you have at your disposal.

When you sit in a slumped posture with your back rounded or bent to one side, the measurable distance between the top of your head and the bottom of your pelvis is decreased. Your entire torso (which includes your spine) is compressed. When you sit up straight with your lower back very arched, your torso will also be compressed, though not to the same degree. However, if you sit in such a way that the normal curves in your spine are maintained but not exaggerated, and your torso muscles work only the amount necessary to keep you upright, your torso will achieve its true functional length. Think of your entire torso—back, front, sides —lengthening up.

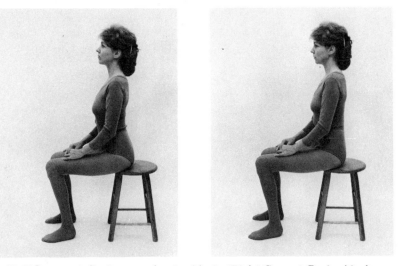

(Left) **Incorrect: Back narrowing (arching).** *(Right)* **Correct: Back widening.**

Torso widening is a concept that should be used along with that of lengthening. If you think only of lengthening, you will probably arch your lower back, thereby narrowing it and actually shortening your spine. To prevent back-arching, think of your lower back widening as you let go of the muscle tension that is causing the arching. Compare the figures on the previous page. The concept of widening is also applicable to the shoulders. You can counteract the tendency to be round-shouldered by thinking of widening across the front of your torso at shoulder level.

For some of you the idea of widening the torso may seem unappealing. Let me assure you that because the torso has greater flexibility along its length than along its width, the overall visual effect of lengthening and widening will be that you appear thinner, not wider.

Combining Concepts I and II

The first two Concepts—*neck free, head forward and up* and *torso lengthening and widening*—are interdependent, with the first helping to bring about the second. As you become more familiar with them, you will find it easier to put them together into one thought, as I will be teaching you to do throughout the book. For example, you can think of your head leading your torso (or spine) into length, or of your head and spine lengthening up. If you are lying down or bending forward, you can think of lengthening out through the top of your head, or, again, of your head leading your spine into length.

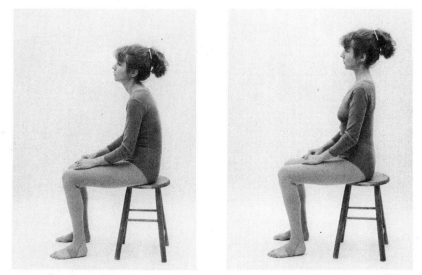

(Left) **Incorrect: Head back and down, spine compressed.** *(Right)* **Correct: Head forward and up, spine lengthening.**

Practicing Concepts I and II

I want you to apply these two Concepts to sitting. Since most people lean against the back of the chair for support, I will show you how to do so correctly. I will then show you how to sit correctly without using any back support other than that provided by your own torso muscles.

Sitting with Back Support. Stop your reading for a moment and examine the way you are sitting. How is your head balanced on top of your neck? How much tension do you have in your neck muscles? Are you sitting in a slump and therefore compressing your back? Or are you sitting straight, but *still* compressing your back because of increased tension and arching in your lower back?

If you decide to make a change in the way you are sitting, mentally instruct your body by using the first two Concepts *before* actually moving. Thinking first will enable you to eliminate the muscle tensions associated with your usual way of sitting so that the corrections you make will last longer.

Think of the first two concepts in the following way: *Let your neck release to let your head balance forward and up, to let your torso lengthen and widen.* As you release your neck muscles, think of your head easing up off your neck and guiding your torso upwards into length.

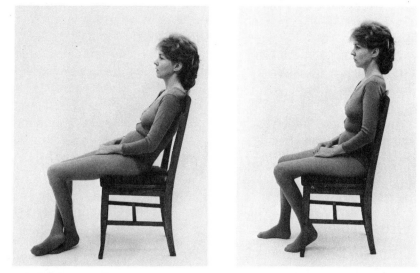

(Left) Incorrect: Slumping against back of chair. *(Right)* Correct: Torso lengthening against back of chair.

Now adjust the way you are sitting so that it is more consistent with the instructions you just gave yourself. If you were sitting in a slumped posture, move your hips all the way back in the chair so your spine can be more upright as you lean against the back of the chair. You may be tempted, as you lengthen your torso, to over-work your back muscles. To avoid doing so, think of your entire back *widening* and see how much tension you can eliminate from your back muscles without losing length in your spine.

Notice that I am not instructing you to relax your muscles—muscles must work when we are sitting up or moving around. The concept of *releasing* will help you eliminate unnecessary muscle tension and at the same time allow your muscles to work only the amount necessary for sitting correctly.

Sitting without Back Support. A good training and strengthening activity for the back is to practice sitting correctly without back support for brief periods. Do not be surprised if you get un-comfortable rather quickly. It will take time for your back to de-velop the endurance to remain lengthened for longer periods with-out support.

Sit on a firm chair close to the front edge. Place both feet on the floor about twelve inches apart. Since your back is unsupported you may be tempted to slump, but don't give in. Instead, *think of your head leading up and your torso lengthening and widening* as you use your back muscles as much as necessary to achieve your true spinal length. If you are sitting correctly, your "sit-bones" (actually, the ischial tuberosities, those two bony prominences at the very bottom of your pelvis) will be pointing directly downward into the seat of the chair.

The way you can identify the correct position for these bones is to put a hand under each buttock directly under each sit-bone and do the following:

Incorrect: Go into a slump and you will feel the sit-bones move forward.

Incorrect: Arch your back and you will feel the sit-bones lift off the chair in back.

Correct: Lengthen and widen your torso and you will feel the sit-bones pointing directly down into your hands.

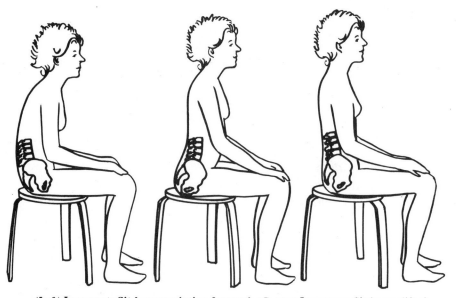

(Left) **Incorrect: Sit-bones pointing forward.** *(Center)* **Incorrect: Sit-bones lifted up in back.** *(Right)* **Correct: Sit-bones pointing straight down.**

Some people think of sitting as simply collapsing. Here is an image that has helped many of my patients overcome that association. Picture yourself "standing" on your sit-bones and let your body sense the verticality of your head, neck, and torso — the same elegant verticality you would have if you were standing.

The wonderful uprightness we humans possess and enjoy is our evolutionary heritage. Our skeletons have evolved over millions of years to allow extremely efficient vertical alignment to take place. Our ability to achieve such good alignment, however, can be defeated by bad furniture, as well as by good furniture used poorly.

Our skeletal muscles work in opposing partnership with one another. For example, the muscles in front of the torso work in partnership with those in back. When you sit with your torso lengthening and widening, all the pairs of muscles that surround the torso can do their job of keeping you upright in a balanced, efficient manner. But when you sit in a slumped posture, your back muscles are overstretched while those in front are overshortened. Neither group can give good support.

CONCEPTS III AND IV

Concept III: Allow Your Legs To Release Away from Your Pelvis

Again, examine the way you are sitting. This time I want you to be aware of any unnecessary tension you may have in the muscles around your hip joints and in your legs.

To locate your hip joints, stand and raise one knee up in front. Notice where the crease occurs in front of the pelvis. You can feel the same crease when sitting.

The Concept of Good Use for the hip joints and legs is to *allow the legs to release away from the pelvis*. When the strong muscles that extend from the hips to the legs are held tight, they interfere with your using the hip joints freely and therefore cause strain in the lower back. Take a moment to release these muscles by thinking of your legs releasing away from your pelvis.

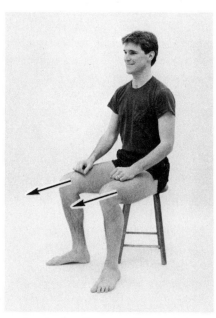

Legs releasing away from pelvis.

You may notice now that you can adjust your sitting to get more length in your spine because the released hip muscles allow your pelvis to be in better alignment with the rest of your torso.

Concept IV: Allow Your Shoulders To Release Out to the Sides

Now that you have lengthened and widened your torso, your shoulders are already on their way to being better balanced. Shoulder placement depends largely upon how well the spine is aligned.

You may be tempted to hold your shoulders back or otherwise consciously adjust the way they are placed, but please do not do so. Instead, renew your thought to *let your head balance forward and up and your torso lengthen and widen*, and then give yourself the instruction to *let your shoulders release out to the sides*. As your shoulder muscles release, your shoulder balance will improve.

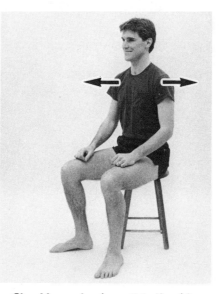

Shoulders releasing out to the sides.

HOW TO "THINK" THE CONCEPTS OF GOOD USE

The best way to apply these Concepts to yourself is to think them as you go about your daily activities. Some people believe they can be mentally in touch with their bodies more effectively with their eyes closed. But I want you to keep them open. Getting accustomed to thinking the Concepts with your eyes open is extremely important because that is how you normally perform most activities (driving, eating dinner, working at your desk, etc.), and thus will be easier for you to integrate them into your daily life.

In addition to applying the Concepts to daily activities, it is a good idea to spend ten to twenty minutes lying down with your eyes closed while you review them mentally. Many of my patients have found this a good way of resting their backs in the middle of the day or of eliminating muscle tension and discomfort before going to sleep.

CHANGING YOUR SELF-IMAGE: AN ADDED BENEFIT

Our postural habits are not only companions to our musculo-skeletal structure, they reflect how we feel about ourselves — our self-image. A change in postural habits requires a change in thought, and the Concepts of Good Use will help you make that change.

Since these Concepts are harmonious with the structure of the body, they enhance the ease with which the body moves. Many of my patients have found they discard negative attitudes toward themselves, such as believing they are clumsy or uncoordinated, as their ability to apply the Concepts of Good Use to daily life increases.

4

Neck Pain

"Take the Weight of Your Head Off Your Neck"

TIGHTENING THE NECK MUSCLES, with the accompanying spinal compression, is one of the most common causes of neck pain. You will understand why this is so after you have allowed me to take you gently into the world of anatomy. Everything you will learn about your body will be relevant to your getting better and staying better.

If you have never studied anatomy, the material will, of course, be new. If you have, the material may seem new because of its specific relevance to alignment, balance, and everyday use. We will begin at the top of the skeletal structure because of the importance of correct head balance on the well-being of the neck and back.

ANATOMY FOR DAILY LIVING

Skeletal Structure of the Head and Neck

On top of your spine sits your head, a not insignificant object weighing about twelve pounds. The part of your spine on which this considerable weight must balance is a very flexible structure, your neck. The bones of your spine are called *vertebrae*; the ones at the top are smaller than those at the bottom. Notice the relative delicacy of the upper neck vertebrae compared to the size of the head. Also notice that the neck has a normal forward curve. The size of this curve varies from person to person.

The vertebrae in the neck are shaped to allow a lot of movement. Emerging from between them on each side are the nerves that go to the shoulders, arms, and hands. The neck also contains many joints, ligaments, spinal discs, and muscles.

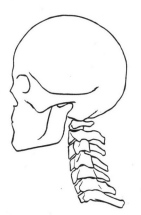

With only the anatomical structures shown in the illustration, your head could not possibly stay balanced upright on your neck. What is missing from this drawing are the neck muscles, whose job is to keep the head poised on top of the neck. Recall how the head falls off balance as soon as the neck muscles relax when someone goes to sleep sitting in a chair.

Muscles in the Back of the Neck

Although all the neck muscles play a role in keeping the head balanced, those in the back of the neck are stronger than the ones in front, and they are most frequently responsible for incorrect head balance. Feel the vertebrae in your neck by walking your fingertips up the back of your neck. Now feel the muscles on each side of these vertebrae. They may feel tight and sore.

When the muscles in the back of the neck become tense and short, they pull the head off balance by taking it *back and down* onto the neck. Compare the two figures below, and notice how the neck becomes compressed when these muscles are shortened.

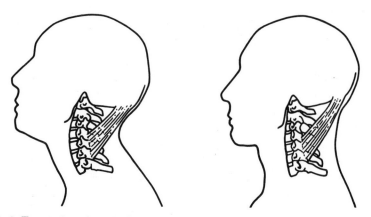

(Left) **Tense, short muscles in back of the neck pull the head back and down.**
(Right) **Released neck muscles allow the head to balance forward and up.**

Among the important muscles in this area are the *suboccipitals*, a group of small, deep muscles that extend from right under the back of the head to the top vertebrae of the neck (below). You can help reduce neck compression by thinking of them as a hand gently supporting the back of your head up off your neck.

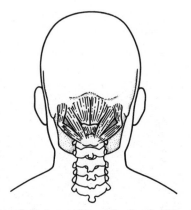

Suboccipital muscles under back of head.

Also important is the *trapezius*, a large muscle that drapes like a cape from the base of the skull out to the shoulders and down the back. You can feel your trapezius by gently pressing your fingertips into the back of your neck, the top of your shoulders, and between your shoulder blades.

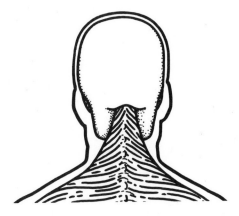

Upper part of trapezius connecting head and shoulders.

When your head is pulled back and down and your shoulders are hunched up, you are overworking the upper fibers of the trapezius. The result can be tenderness and spasm. As you learn to release the trapezius so that your head and shoulders can balance correctly, the discomfort you have in this muscle will decrease.

Skeletal Poise of the Head

Because the head is heavy and is perched on the very top of the spine, it affects the well-being of the entire spine. Just as incorrect use of your head can compress your spine, correct use can help your spine lengthen. Many of my patients ask how this spinal lengthening is possible. The answer lies in the way the head is balanced on the neck.

If you were to balance a human skull on two fingertips (to simulate the way it rests on top of the neck), it would immediately roll forward because it has more weight in front of the head-neck pivot point than in back. In other words, the head is not placed squarely on top of the neck. I like to think of the head as being "elegantly unbalanced."

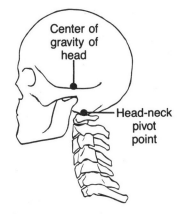

The "elegantly unbalanced" head.

The strong muscles in the back of the neck counterbalance the weight of the head. When they are kept too short as they do their counterbalancing work, they compress the neck, force the neck out of good alignment with the rest of the spine, and cause the entire spine to shorten. These harmful conditions disappear when the muscles in back work at their optimum length—a length that allows good spacing between the vertebrae, a centered alignment of the head and neck with the rest of the spine, and free movement.

Achieving beneficial head balance is a matter of eliminating unnecessary muscle tension, of *not interfering* with the body's wonderful design. Since the head is heavier in front, it will automatically rotate out of its backward tilt when the muscles in back are allowed to release and lengthen. All the neck muscles can then work efficiently in concert, and the entire spine will be able to lengthen.

Young children provide a wonderful example of correct head balance as they sit, run, and climb. When they grow older, tension in the neck muscles interferes with this balance, with the result that the spine becomes increasingly compressed, setting the stage for neck and back problems.

LEARNING CORRECT HEAD BALANCE

Since the health of the nerves, discs, joints, and muscles of
your neck depends upon how efficiently the weight of your head
is managed, you need to be able to tell the difference between
correct and incorrect head balance. As you read, you can begin to
explore this difference.

Incorrect Head Balance

You must be able to recognize the incorrect "back and down"
use of the head in order to avoid it, so I want you to feel it on
yourself again, as you did in Chapter 3. Place one hand on the
back of your neck with the side of your little finger directly under
your head. Now tighten the muscles under your hand so that your
head is pulled back and down. Repeat this motion a few times,
picturing how the structures in the back of your neck are being
compressed.

Few people realize that when they look straight ahead while
sitting slumped, the head is actually being pulled back and down
on the neck in exactly this same way. Compare how the head is
balanced in the figures below. Besides compressing the neck,
incorrect head balance causes the head and neck to be held too far
in front of the shoulders. This incorrect alignment can increase
the prominent "bump" some people get at the base of the neck.

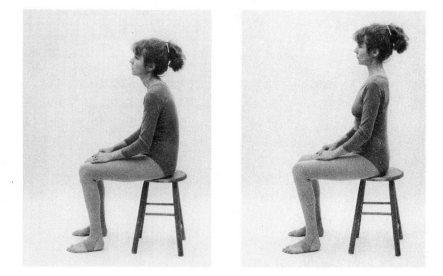

Correct Head Balance

To correct your head balance you will be applying the first two Concepts of Good Use:

Allow your neck muscles to release so that your head can balance forward and up.
Allow your torso to release into length and width.

Look again at the drawings of tense muscles and released muscles in the back of the neck (page 31) and try to visualize the muscles in the back of your own neck. Allow your muscles to release so they can get longer, and at the same time adjust the way you are sitting to give your spine more length (be sure not to tilt your head back). If you are starting this correction from a slumped position, the back of your head will lift up slightly and your nose will lower. Now place your hand on the back of your neck. You may find that your neck feels longer and that your head is not displaced as far in front of your shoulders as it was.

Do not try to find a correct position for your head—there is no such thing. The idea of positioning the head is too confining, and it will make your neck tense. Instead, think of correct head *balance* and of your head being able to move freely on the very top of your neck. Practice looking around while maintaining spinal length.

APPLYING CORRECT HEAD BALANCE

I am now going to guide you into using correct head balance for the routine head motions you use many times a day. Before practicing, be sure your entire spine is lengthening. It is impossible to balance and use your head correctly while you are sitting in a slumped posture.

Looking Down

If you are like most people and spend many hours a day looking down at your work (reading, typing, sewing, etc.), the way your head and neck are aligned can either injure or help your neck.

The most common mistake people make is to drop the head and neck down toward their work, thereby pulling the neck out of alignment with the rest of the spine. Collapsing over your work is not necessary and is detrimental to the structures of the neck. Compare the following two pictures:

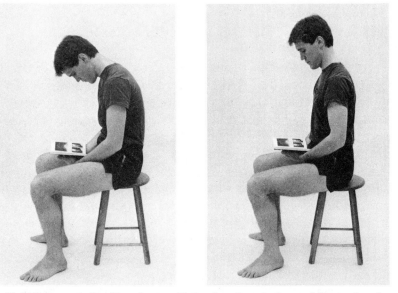

(Left) Incorrect: Looking down with head and neck dropped forward; spine compressed. *(Right)* Correct: Looking down with head and spine lengthening up.

To look down correctly, release the muscles in the back of your neck sufficiently to let your head simply *tilt forward.* While looking down, you should continue thinking of your entire head releasing up off your neck and your spine lengthening. Practice tilting your head forward a few times by looking straight ahead and then down at this book.

You may find that the habit of dropping your head, neck, and shoulders forward over your work is so strong that just the thought of looking down starts your upper body moving downwards. If so, you need to apply Alexander's process of *inhibition* (see Chapter 3) to yourself in the following way: once you have made the decision to look down, delay doing so for a moment in order to give yourself time to replace the impulse to slump forward with that of *lengthening.* By pausing briefly before carrying out a familiar activity, you will give your body the opportunity to be guided by the Concepts of Good Use.

I want you to feel for yourself how looking down correctly affects your neck. Start by looking straight ahead and place the fingertips of one hand vertically along the back of your neck. Now tilt your head downward, and feel with your fingers how the back of your neck becomes gently stretched, providing beneficial traction to all its structures.

Looking Up

You may be wondering whether it is always wrong to tilt the head back. No. It is natural to do for certain purposes, such as looking up above eye level or stretching. Tilting the head back becomes detrimental only when you do it repeatedly as a postural habit.

The mistake most people make when they look up is that in doing so they compress the entire spine. Even when maintaining length in the spine, looking up can be hard on the delicate structures of the neck. To protect them, think of your entire spine lengthening up to help support your head.

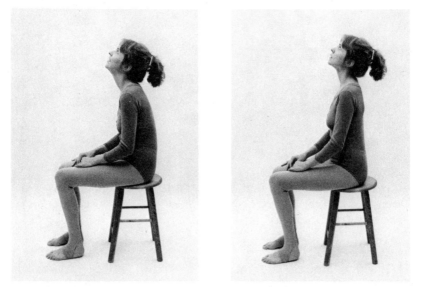

(Left) Incorrect: Looking up with spine compressed. *(Right)* Correct: Looking up with spine lengthening.

Practice looking at the ceiling without losing the length in your spine. As you return to looking straight ahead or down, give extra thought to releasing the muscles in the back of your neck. Tilting your head back requires you to shorten these muscles, so you want to release that shortening when you no longer need it. Here again, if the thought of looking up starts your body going into a postural slump, pause for a moment and think of your entire torso lengthening upwards.

Looking to the Side

Incorrect head turning causes a great deal of neck compression. The mistake most people make is to pull the head back and down and compress the spine. (You should only tilt your head back when looking to the side above eye level.) Compare the two photographs:

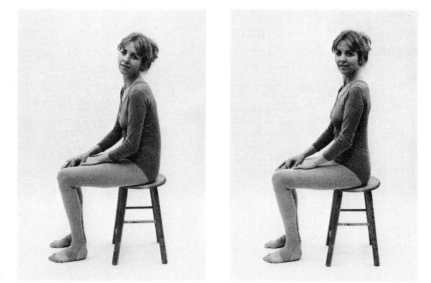

(Left) **Incorrect: Looking to the side with head pulled back and down, spine compressed.** *(Right)* **Correct: Looking to the side with head balancing forward and up, spine lengthening.**

Practice turning your head a few times while releasing the muscles in the back of your neck and lengthening your spine. Turning your head without pulling it backwards will feel strange at first, even though you did it exactly this way when you were a small child. (Children turn their heads correctly until they develop the habit of slumping.)

Should you ever wake up in the morning with a stiff neck, you will find you can turn your head much farther with less pain if you do it correctly.

After practicing these three ways of using your head and neck with greater ease, you should become aware of performing simple daily activities with less tension in your neck. This will, of necessity, slow you down. However, by taking time to examine how you move, you will gradually be able to eliminate detrimental habits of use and develop beneficial ones.

Coping with Eyeglasses

Anyone who wears glasses may occasionally find them a hindrance to using the head and neck correctly. For example, if your glasses fit too loosely, you may develop the habit of pulling your head back to keep them from sliding off. Have them adjusted as often as necessary to fit securely.

I wear bifocals and find that they are sometimes a problem. When I read at eye level or above, which occurs when I look at a bulletin board or browse in a bookstore, the glasses force me to tilt my head back to see through the reading section at the bottom of the lenses. I minimize the strain of this position by maintaining length in my spine as I tilt my head back to read. When I am finished, I lengthen the back of my neck by releasing the neck muscles and looking down briefly.

Bifocals that have their reading sections just a bit too high or too low for your most common reading position can also cause poor head-neck use. If you have neck pain when you read, you may be able to solve the problem by having your bifocals re-aligned.

Some people need to have "occupational lenses" made for special situations. I met a man — a bifocal wearer — whose work required him to alternate between reading above eye level and reading at table level. He eliminated the need to keep tilting his head back by getting double bifocals: each lens has a small reading section at the bottom and another at the top. The middle section is for distance vision.

If you wear reading glasses or bifocals for close work, but also need to see comfortably and clearly at the distance required by some other activity, such as working at a computer or reading music at the piano, you may need to have a special pair of glasses made for that viewing distance. The right glasses will give you better vision while allowing you to maintain good head-neck-torso alignment.

APPLICATION TO SPECIFIC MEDICAL PROBLEMS

The delicate structures of the neck are so vulnerable to wear and tear from poor postural habits that sometimes medical problems result or existing problems can worsen. Improved daily use of your head and neck can aid recovery.

Pinched Nerves

Pinched nerves in the neck frequently cause pain in the shoulder, arm, or hand. If you have such pain and your physician has determined that it originates in your neck, then correct use of your head and neck is essential.

A nerve is most likely to become pinched when the space between two vertebrae is made smaller by spinal compression, often caused by misuse of the strong muscles in the back of the neck. Keeping these muscles longer and more released allows more space for the nerves, so that the pain diminishes or disappears.

One patient discovered, during his first Alexander lesson, that he could turn his pain on and off like a faucet. When he pulled his head back and down, he felt pain in his hand; when he let his head release forward and up, the pain stopped.

Arthritis

Osteoarthritis is the most common type of arthritis and is thought to be associated with normal aging. Osteoarthritis in the neck responds well to improved use by becoming less painful and restrictive. Since tension in the neck muscles imposes more restriction on the involved joints, reducing this tension allows more joint motion to take place.

Osteophytes, or bone spurs (a characteristic of osteoarthritis) cause many people a great deal of pain. The body deposits extra calcium on bones where there is excessive pressure and stress. Therefore, you will benefit more from physical therapy or other treatment for this condition by learning to reduce compression and muscle tension in your neck. You may also help prevent the formation of more bone spurs.

Neck Tension

A major cause of neck pain is chronic tension in the neck muscles. Prolonged muscle tension irritates the muscle fibers and eventually causes the muscles to go into spasm.

If this is the cause of your pain, you probably tense your neck muscles every time you talk on the phone, work at your desk, or drive your car. You may feel that you cannot perform these activities with less tension, but let me assure you that just as your thoughts can cause muscle tension, your thoughts can also tell that tension to go away. Increased awareness of correct head balance will enable you to identify and change tension patterns that eventually lead to pain.

Tension Headache

Headaches originating from tense neck muscles are common. They can be caused by long periods of faulty head-neck-torso alignment while you bend over your work, or they can be caused by emotional stress. You are already learning to correct the first cause.

The second—tensing the neck muscles in response to emotional stress—is more difficult to eliminate. Here is a recommendation that might help. Alexander's Concepts of Good Use provide an excellent way for you to identify inappropriate muscle tension. When you feel your neck muscles responding to a stressful situation in the way that usually results in a tension headache, use the Concepts to reduce tension throughout your entire body. You may be able to prevent a painful headache from developing.

Whiplash Injury

A whiplash injury occurs when the head is forcefully and quickly thrown forward and back, traumatizing the structures in the neck. Car accidents are the most common cause. If you have had this type of injury, any treatment you are receiving will be much more effective when you learn to release your neck muscles and keep your spine in good alignment.

The pain from a whiplash injury often creates a vicious pain-tension cycle. The pain causes muscle tension, which causes more pain, which causes more tension. By learning to reduce tension in your neck muscles, you can prevent the cycle from beginning.

After a serious neck injury you have to be constantly on guard so that you do not re-injure yourself. It is difficult, and borders on the absurd, to try to treat a neck injury without dealing with the entire spine. A whiplash injury can so severely damage the delicate structures of the neck that they have no tolerance for incorrect spinal alignment, which may occur at any time. You could be doing something as routine as brushing your teeth or talking on the phone.

If you have had a whiplash injury, read the information in the following two chapters for help in using your entire spine and shoulders correctly.

An Overstraightened Neck

A neck that is too straight is not as common as one that is too curved, but it can be just as painful.

Some people have very straight necks simply as an inherited spinal characteristic. Others bring about the condition with the postural habit of pulling the chin into the front of the neck. I have also seen necks that have become too straight in people addicted to doing too many Yoga shoulder stands, an exercise that over-stretches the muscles and ligaments in the back of the neck until they no longer give proper support.

The curves of the spine are extremely important and should not be flattened out. If your neck is too straight, using your neck freely (with less muscle tension) for all normal motions will restore your head and neck to a dynamically balanced state. You should also be doing exercises that gently restore the normal mobility of your spine (see Chapter 11).

5
Low Back Pain

"The Waist Is Not a Hinge"

THE LOWER BACK AREA of the torso is deserving of our deepest sympathies because it is the most common site of back pain. The torso is a structural triumph providing both flexibility and strength; however, it can only serve us properly when used in a well-integrated way.

You may already know that your postural habits and ways of moving are harmful to your back. They will be easier to improve once you understand the relationship between how your lower back is structured and the way it should be used.

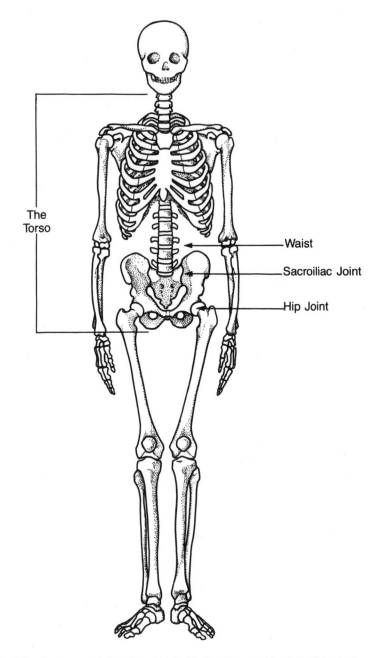

The
Torso

Waist

Sacroiliac Joint

Hip Joint

Think of the torso as one functional unit. Notice the considerable distance between the waist and the hip joints.

ANATOMY FOR DAILY LIVING

The Torso

I want you to start thinking of your torso as *one functional unit*. The drawing on the opposite page will help you visualize it in this way. The waist area of the torso is flexible, but it is not designed as a hinge and therefore should not be used as one.

Like the unicorn, the waist is a mythical creature. It exists as a concept, but we get into trouble when we think of the waist as a real entity, with hinge-like qualities. Such faulty thinking leads to faulty use, and faulty use of the waist is responsible for many lower back problems.

There is nothing wrong with using the flexibility of your spine when it is appropriate, such as for dancing, exercising, or engaging in sports. But your back can be injured when you *misuse* its flexibility. It should not be misused by bending from the waist or by slumping, which keeps the waist bent continually.

Perhaps you have heard of the sacroiliac joints, which connect the bottom of the spine to the pelvis. This connection is a very secure one and does not allow for much movement. When you slump or bend from the waist you are putting strain on the many ligaments that go across the sacroiliac joints.

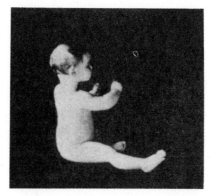

This photograph of an eight-month-old baby exemplifies the structural unity of the torso. When you were a baby you also used to sit in this beautiful way. Notice how the entire torso (spine, pelvis, and shoulders) is in good alignment. Also notice how this baby's head is poised on her neck: the back of her head is coming up off her neck instead of pressing down on it (as it does when we slump), and her whole spine is lengthening.

The Hip Joints

The hip joints are where your legs join your torso. In contrast to the much less flexible sacroiliac joints, the hip joints permit a great deal of free movement because of their ball and socket design. As you are reading, move your knees apart and together. You can also roll your thighs in and out, or raise a knee up toward your chest. All these motions are taking place in your hip joints.

You may be surprised at how far below the waist area the hip joints really are. Turn back to the illustration of the skeleton. It will help you visualize this distance more easily. To feel your hip joints' approximate location on yourself when sitting, place your fingertips on the front bones of your pelvis — those prominent bony points on each side — and then slide your fingers slightly down and in until they meet the crease of your legs. Your fingers are now pointing down into your hip joints.

The hip joints are surrounded by many powerful muscles. When these muscles are held tight, they pull the pelvis out of correct alignment with the rest of the torso, which strains the lower back. Therefore, it is extremely important for those of you with low back pain to use your hip joints freely.

Take a moment to do a brief visualization exercise. Picture yourself standing, then mentally divide your body into upper and lower halves. Did you divide yourself at the waist? Most people do, even though skeletally and functionally the waist is the wrong place for such a division. From now on, should you indulge in such imagery, I want you to think of yourself as being divided into upper and lower halves at your *hip joints* rather than your waist.

The Spine

Among the components of the spine are the vertebrae (the bones of the spine), discs, ligaments, nerve roots, and facet joints.

Spinal Discs. Separating the vertebrae from one another are the spinal discs. They have a fibrous outer shell and a soft, gelatinous substance in the center. Their functions are to bear weight, act as shock absorbers, and, because they are flexible, enhance spinal movement. The discs are located in the front part of the spine, that is, in front of the spinal cord and nerve roots.

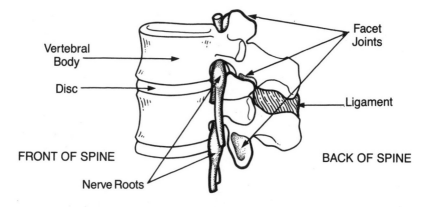

The spinal discs are particularly vulnerable to poor postural habits. When a disc is described as "bulging," part of it has protruded backwards toward the spinal cord and nerve roots. A *herniated* disc is one in which the gelatinous inner substance has partially or completely broken through the fibrous outer wall; again, the protrusion is backwards toward the spinal cord and nerve roots. Being able to visualize what happens when a disc misbehaves will help you avoid harmful postural habits that lead to disc problems.

Compare the drawings below. On the right is a disc being distorted by pressure. Such distortion occurs often and is not harmful unless it continues *in one direction* for long periods of time, which happens when you slump. Continual slumping may gradually force part of a disc in the lower back backwards and out toward the spinal cord and nerve roots. Even if slumping does not actually cause the disc to herniate, it may so weaken the back wall of the disc that bending forward from the waist one time too many does the final job.

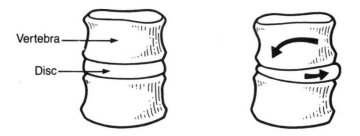

(Left) Disc in neutral position. *(Right)* Disc being distorted by pressure.

There are two common anxiety-provoking misconceptions about spinal discs that I want to dispel:

1. Some people become very anxious when they are told they have a "slipped" disc, because they imagine the disc as an unattached object that can slide all over the place. The term "slipped" is misleading and inaccurate: discs do not slip around like a piece of wet soap. Part of their substance can bulge or herniate out where it does not belong, but the spinal discs are very securely attached to the vertebrae above and below.

2. Some people worry about being able to feel their spinal discs with their fingers. Reach behind you and touch your spine. What you are feeling are the backs of the vertebrae and the muscles on each side, but not the discs, which are much farther forward. You cannot reach the discs nor feel them from outside the body even if they have bulged or herniated.

Facet Joints. The vertebrae are connected to each other in back by small gliding joints called *facet joints.* The facet joints contribute to the flexibility of the spine. When the lower back is habitually arched more than it should be, these little joints carry more body weight than they should and become compressed. The extra weight eventually irritates them sufficiently to cause pain, damage their delicate structure, and decrease their flexibility.

Therefore, how you align your spine during all your daily activities strongly influences the health of your spinal facet joints. When your entire torso is kept in good alignment by lengthening and widening, the weight borne by the lower spine falls where it belongs: on the front part of the vertebrae and on the discs, not on the facet joints.

Spinal Ligaments. Ligaments are strong, flexible strips of tissue that lie across all the joints in the body and attach directly to the bones close to the joints. Like a checkrein, they prevent excessive joint motion that could damage the delicate joint structures.

The spinal column gets much of its stability and support from ligaments. Some are long, traversing the entire length of the spine, and others are short, extending from one vertebra to its neighbor above or below.

Our daily postural habits affect the well-being of our spinal ligaments. A slumped sitting posture gradually overstretches the ligaments in the lower back until they can no longer give effective support.

The Abdominal Muscles

The lower back has no greater friend than these impressive—but often inadequately used—muscles. The abdominal muscles are a natural corset because they are perfectly constructed to give support. No matter how dissatisfied you may be with the performance of your abdominals, let me assure you that they are capable of doing a good job. Even if you have had abdominal surgery, these amazing muscles can be strengthened and trained to support your back properly.

The abdominal muscles come in layers, and what is most remarkable is that each layer gives support in a different direction from the other layers. The result is very similar to a four-way-stretch corset. The commonly used term "stomach muscles" is misleading because these muscles cover a much larger area than just the stomach. Later in this chapter (and in Chapter 11, which contains a daily exercise program), I will teach you how to train your abdominal muscles to work more efficiently.

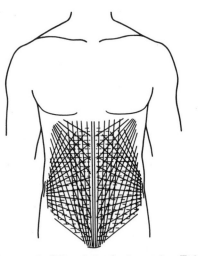

The different lines of support of the abdominal muscles. Think of a four-way-stretch corset.

LEARNING CORRECT USE OF THE LOWER BACK

A good way to learn to use your lower back correctly is with an activity you do many times a day. Alexander always started his lessons by working with people as they got in and out of a chair. I am going to do the same with you.

You will need a straight chair and a long mirror. Place the chair sideways to the mirror so you can see yourself in profile. Sit toward the front edge, which will make it easier for you to move correctly while you are learning, and will allow you to see the alignment of your lower back. (Once you are familiar with the correct way of moving, you can sit all the way back in the chair.)

Change your sitting alignment, if necessary, so that your torso has more length. If you find you are now arching your back, reduce the arch by allowing that area to release into width while still maintaining length in your spine. Notice that I am not telling you to keep your back straight. The instruction to "keep straight" would make your muscles more tense and painful and prevent you from moving freely.

Remember, the spine is *not* straight; it is normally curved and flexible. There are times when the spine should be more "straightly" aligned, such as when you are sitting, and times when its flexibility should be used, such as when you are exercising. The concept of lengthening will help you achieve correct alignment of your spine for all activities.

And now think to yourself the first three Concepts of Good Use:

Allow your neck muscles to release so that your head can balance forward and up.
Allow your torso to release into length and width.
Allow your legs to release away from your pelvis.

Do not start moving yet. Sit quietly a moment while repeating the Concepts a few times to give your body a chance to be influenced by them when you do start to move.

Seeing Correct Use in the Mirror

Lean forward a few times without actually standing up, while continuing to think of your head leading your spine into length and your legs releasing away from your pelvis. Pay particular attention to the alignment of your lower back, being sure not to lean from the waist. Also be sure that you are not arching your back. Look at the photographs, and look in the mirror to see that you are leaning forward correctly. (Turning your head to look in the mirror will not interfere with lengthening your spine).

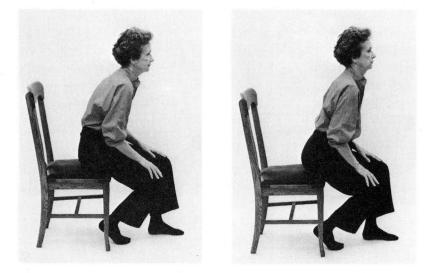

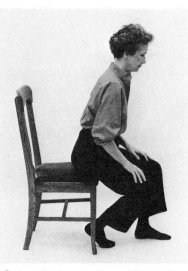

(Top left) Incorrect: Lower back rounding while getting out of a chair. *(Top right)* Incorrect: Lower back arching. *(Bottom)* Correct: Torso lengthening and widening. The head is leading the torso into length.

Now stand up and sit down a few times. If you find that you are starting to round or arch your back in your old, habitual way, delay moving for a moment and deliberately put aside the decision to stand or sit.

Focus your thoughts on the Concepts of Good Use and continue to think about them as you move. In this way, you will learn to inhibit your usual body response to standing or sitting. Move slowly, looking in the mirror to be sure your spine stays in correct alignment. Do not be surprised if your legs feel as if they are working harder than usual. This is a good sign. An important side benefit of using your back correctly is that your legs become stronger.

Feeling Correct Use

I want you to feel the action of your back muscles with your own hands. Again, sit close to the front edge of the chair and place the fingers of both hands gently on the muscles on each side of your spine at waist level. Lean forward (without getting up yet) and feel your spinal muscles as you try three different ways of moving.

Incorrect: Lean forward from the waist. The spinal muscles in the lower back do not work at all.

Incorrect: Arch your back while leaning forward. The spinal muscles shorten and work too hard, compressing the structures of your lower back. You will feel the muscles contract and bunch up as your back arches.

Correct: Lean forward while allowing your torso to lengthen and widen and your hip joints to move freely. The spinal muscles are releasing and working efficiently to maintain correct spinal alignment. You will feel the muscles contract but they will not bunch up the way they do when you arch your back.

Remove your fingers from your back and lean forward the correct way until your weight is over your feet and you can stand up easily. Stand up and sit down a few times while checking yourself in the mirror. Be sure to think of your head leading your spine into length just before you move and while you are moving. By seeing what correct use looks like in the mirror, and by feeling correct use with your fingers, you will gradually gain the skills necessary for using your back in a way that lets it heal and stay strong.

Start applying what you have just learned to the many times you stand up and sit down. Be sure to check yourself in a mirror occasionally. You may find it helpful to practice with a friend, so you can correct each other.

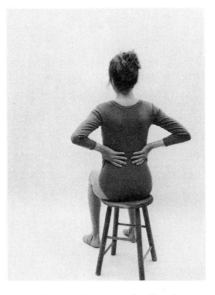

Place your fingers over the muscles on each side of your spine so you can feel them working as you lean forward.

APPLICATION TO DAILY ACTIVITIES

Even though we are dealing primarily with the lower back in this chapter, when you practice using your back correctly you should also be aware of your head and neck. Correct use of the entire head-neck-torso unit is needed to help any one painful area.

As you work with the following instructions, it may seem as though there is a great deal to keep in mind for such simple activities as standing, walking, or bending. You will soon realize, however, that most of the instructions are the same ones you have been learning. Such repetition is necessary if you are to change the postural habits of many years. Gradually, the new way of moving will become more automatic, and you will not have to think about it so much.

Standing

Correcting the way you stand is extremely important because it is the best way to start training your abdominal muscles to support your back. Perhaps, like many others, you have gone through the following thought sequence: *I have low back pain and should strengthen my abdominal muscles, therefore I must lie down and start doing abdominal muscle exercises.* I have no objection to exercises done lying down, and will be teaching you some in Chapter 11. I only object to the assumption that such exercises *automatically* lead to correct use of the abdominal muscles when you are up and about. Since these muscles must protect your back while you are standing and moving around, they should be trained while you are standing and moving.

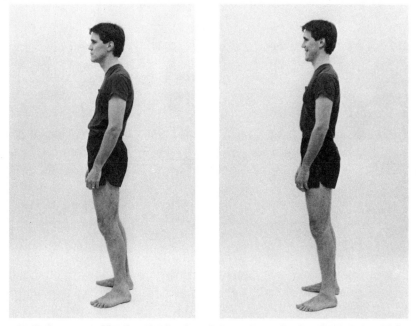

(Left) Incorrect: Head pulled back and down, lower back compressed. *(Right)* Correct: Head releasing forward and up, entire torso lengthening and widening.

Stand in profile to the mirror and check your alignment. Perhaps your back is too arched or your shoulders are too far behind your hips. Look at the photographs, and notice the improvement in your alignment as you apply the first two Concepts of Good Use:

Release the muscles in the back of your neck so that the back of your head can ease up off your neck (you can do this with your head turned sideways to look in the mirror).

Gently lengthen your entire spine, being sure not to pull your head back.

Combine these two corrections into one by thinking of your head leading your spine into length. You may feel your lower abdominal muscles working harder. They are starting to give your lower back the support it needs.

I have been emphasizing the importance of releasing muscles, so it may seem like a contradiction to tell you to work these muscles harder. But remember that released does not mean relaxed. Your abdominal muscles must work hard enough to support your lower back and keep it from arching too much when you are standing. Remember that you do not want to flatten your back completely. The spine needs its normal curves to be efficiently balanced.

Experiment now, while standing, with three ways of using your abdominal muscles. You will discover that you *do* have control over them:

Incorrect: Tighten your abdominal muscles vigorously by pulling them in as hard as you can. Notice how hard it is to breathe.

Incorrect: Relax your abdominal muscles completely. Notice that your entire torso goes into a slump. This means that your spine is losing length and is becoming compressed. It may be less obvious, but this posture also interferes with breathing because the rib cage is compressed.

Correct: Lengthen your entire spine up toward your head and think of *gently* tightening the lower part of your abdominal muscles in the area just below the belly button. Thinking of just the lower area will prevent you from overtightening. Many of my patients find that lengthening the spine automatically results in the lower abdominal muscles working the correct amount.

As your abdominal muscles start to give support, the muscles in the small of your back will be able to release. All the muscles that wrap around your torso will then be doing their job in a more balanced way.

Check your alignment in the mirror: your abdominal muscles should work just enough to decrease the arch in your lower back, which lengthens your spine. Although you may be dependent on your mirror at first, you will gradually begin to sense correct alignment. Start becoming aware of how you stand as you wait for an elevator or stand in line.

Walking

The initial instructions to give yourself while walking are the same as those for standing: *Let your head lead your spine into length.*

Now add the third Concept of Good Use: *Let your legs release away from your pelvis.* I also like to think of my knees leading my legs forward with each step.

Think specifically of releasing your buttock muscles as you walk. Yes, I am telling you to *release* your buttock muscles, not tighten them, even though this advice may directly contradict instructions you received elsewhere. Releasing these muscles is extremely important for the well-being of your lower back (and for the sciatic nerves, as you will learn later).

To clarify this point, let me familiarize you with a major anatomical difference between the abdominal muscles and the buttock muscles. Your abdominal muscles lie on the torso only and do not go to the legs. Therefore, making them work harder supports your back but does not interfere with free leg motion. The buttock muscles, on the other hand, extend from the torso to the legs. Therefore, tightening them interferes with using your legs freely and causes strain in your lower back.

Practice walking while lengthening your spine and releasing your buttock muscles so that your legs swing forward easily. The new ease of movement you will experience may make you feel like prancing! Now try walking with your buttock muscles held tight. See how much more difficut it is to move and how awkward you feel.

Those of you who believe that tightening the buttock muscles will lessen a "heavy" look in the hips and buttocks will find the opposite is true. You can actually look thinner when you release your buttocks because you are also allowing your torso to achieve more length. Many of my patients have been asked by friends if they have lost weight when, in fact, their weight is the same. The difference in how they look is the result of increased spinal length and a more easeful way of moving.

Reaching the Floor

Almost every patient with back trouble has learned the hard way that bending from the waist is painful and harmful. You can reach the floor without hurting your back by partially bending your knees and inclining your torso forward, or by squatting all the way down.

An important part of correct bending or squatting to reach the floor is knowing how to protect your knees. Some people believe that bending the knees can harm them, but I find this hard to accept. We would never have lasted as a species in the jungles of yesteryear if these all-important joints had not proved fine equipment in our struggle to survive. Just watching children at play as they frequently squat and come up again, and knowing that in many cultures elderly people squat with ease, tells us these joints can work efficiently.

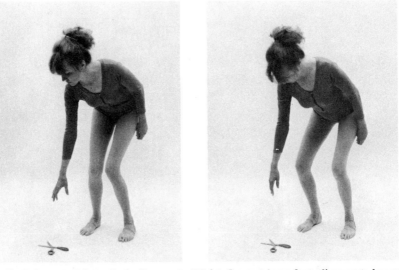

(Left) **Incorrect knee-foot alignment.** *(Right)* **Correct knee-foot alignment: knees bending over tops of feet.**

The problem lies not in the knee bending, but in *how* the bending is done. Whether you squat all the way down or only half-way, the cardinal rule is to keep your knees in line with the tops of your feet. Letting the knees go to the inside or outside of your feet strains your knee joints. Compare the two photographs above, and be sure to use correct knee-foot alignment every time you bend your knees.

If squatting all the way down hurts your knees, or if you have a specific knee problem that has led your physician to restrict their motion, you should bend your knees partially while inclining your torso forward from the hips until you can reach the floor. Be sure to lengthen your back while leaning forward. The photographs below show three correct ways of bending.

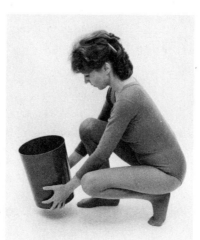

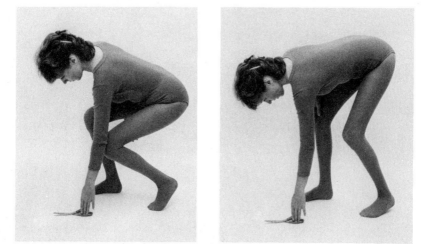

Three correct ways of bending down, showing different amounts of knee bending.

HEELS DOWN OR HEELS UP?

In a discussion of how to squat all the way down, a lively debate often ensues between the "heels down" and "heels up" schools of thought. The fact of the matter is that neither way is right or wrong in itself. You can keep your heels either up or down depending on the task at hand and how you want to affect the alignment of your lower back.

Heels down: Keeping the heels down requires considerable flexibility in the hip, knee, and ankle joints and is, therefore, impossible for some people. With your heels on the floor, you are more stable for long-term squatting, a form of "sitting" in cultures that do not use chairs.

When the heels stay down, the normal forward curve of the lower back is reversed and the weight of the pelvis gently stretches the lower spine (left photo). This traction eases tight back muscles and relieves pressure on the spinal facet joints.

Heels up: Letting the heels come off the floor when squatting allows the head, neck, and torso to stay in a more neutral or centered alignment (right photo). It is, therefore, less disturbing to the structures of the lower back. It is also more practical for quick, easy bending to pick up small objects from the floor.

I usually teach my patients the heels up method because of its practicality and because it is a good strengthening exercise for the back muscles.

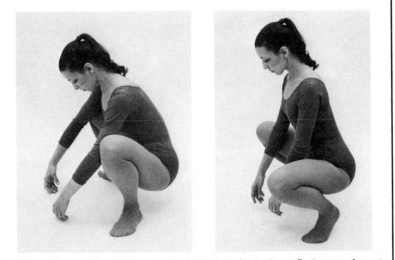

(Left) Squatting with heels down. *(Right)* Squatting with heels up. Both ways of squatting are correct. Notice the different effect each has on alignment of the lower back.

If you like to squat all the way down, here are guidelines for doing so correctly:

1. Place your feet slightly apart and stand quietly for a moment without moving while you release your neck and let your head lead your torso into length.

2. Go into a squat, leaning forward and letting your heels come up off the floor, until you can touch the floor in front of you with your hands. While bending down, be sure to look at the floor, which will help you keep your balance and prevent you from pulling your head back and down. Also, think of your hips, knees, and ankles as free to fold under you.

3. Return to standing by copying the method little children use: lean farther forward so you can put your hands on the floor and give yourself a good boost upwards. Think of lengthening your spine as you stand up.

Squatting and bending correctly may seem difficult at first, but gradually your legs will get stronger and your balance will improve. You can practice while watching yourself sideways in a mirror to see if you are rounding or arching your back.

Bending Halfway Down

Reaching down to take something from a coffee table, to make a bed, or to open a low drawer is more hazardous to the lower back than squatting all the way down because almost everyone bends from the waist and keeps the knees straight. The following pictures illustrate the incorrect way and two correct ways of bending halfway down. Notice that when you bend correctly, the spine stays lengthened and at least one knee is bent.

To practice bending correctly, place a pencil or other small object on a chair and stand in front of the chair as though you were going to pick the object up.

1. Place one foot slightly in front of the other and give yourself the instructions to *release the muscles in the back of your neck and lengthen your spine.*

2. Bend your front knee or both knees and incline your torso forward from your hip joints until you can reach the pencil, making sure not to round your upper back. With only your front knee bent, you have to lean farther forward. If your back feels strained, bend both knees and keep your back more vertical.

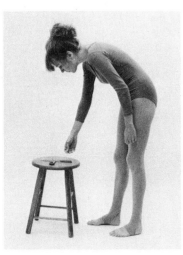

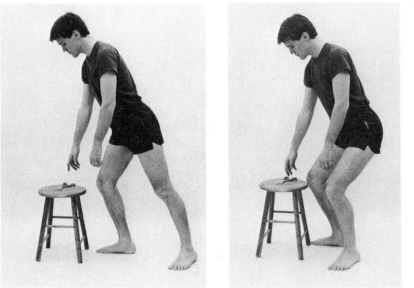

(Top) **Incorrect: Bending from the waist.** *(Bottom left)* **Correct: One knee bent; head leading the torso into length.** *(Bottom right)* **Correct: Both knees bent.**

Practice bending a few times to pick up and replace the pencil. Be sure your knees are bending over the tops of your feet. Whenever you bend correctly, either halfway or all the way down, your back muscles are working and therefore getting stronger. That is why the correct use of your back is actually therapeutic.

Lifting

The instructions for squatting also apply to lifting a heavy object, except that for lifting you should take a wider stance.

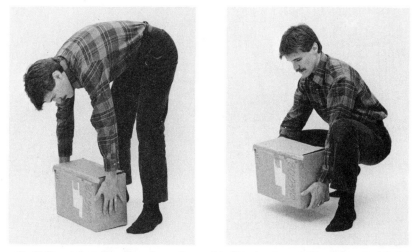

(Left) Incorrect: Bending from the waist. The back could be injured. *(Right)* Correct: Back muscles are working to maintain spinal lengthening. The back is protected.

If you have a history of back trouble, you should avoid lifting altogether. But if you must lift something, be sure to bend from your knees, not your waist, and keep your back lengthened. Stand very close to the object you are lifting, or else do not lift it. You must also be sure your back is not twisted; it should be centered rather than bent to the side or rotated. A centered back is important for any activity requiring strength, such as opening a stuck window or door.

Sitting

Few people realize that sitting incorrectly can slowly but inevitably spell disaster for the lower back. The spine always needs support, which must come either from your own muscles or the chair you are sitting in. Sitting becomes dangerous when you give the job of supporting your back to a poorly designed chair.

There are two ways you can sit in a chair without hurting your back:

1. Sit close to the front edge and use your back muscles to maintain spinal length.

2. Sit all the way back in the seat and use the back of the chair for support. If the chair is too deep, put a firm pillow behind you for proper support.

The mistake most people make is to sit halfway back in the seat and then slump against the back of the chair.

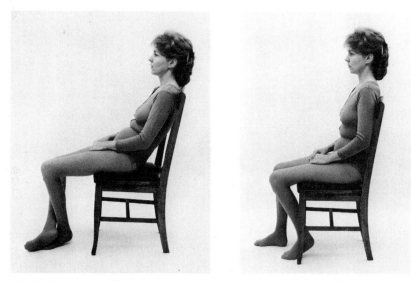

(Left) **Incorrect: Slumping against back of chair.** *(Right)* **Correct: Torso lengthening against back of chair.**

If you must sit on a deep couch, either sit close to the front edge with your back lengthened, or all the way back in the seat, using the back of the couch for support. People with short legs should fold their legs under them when sitting all the way back, provided their legs are flexible enough. Actually, a good rule is to avoid deep couches altogether.

If you are not used to sitting correctly, you will gradually return to slumping. Whenever you notice this happening, just move your hips farther back in the chair and lengthen your spine. You may need to repeat this many times a day until your back develops endurance and sitting correctly becomes more automatic.

Sneezing

I am not being frivolous with this topic because sneezing is serious business for back pain sufferers. The sudden force of a sneeze can actually cause injury to the structures of the spine.

If you are standing when you feel a sneeze coming, bend your knees slightly and brace or support your back by placing one hand on your thigh or a table near you. This will stabilize your back and prevent injury. If you are sitting, support your back by putting one hand on your thigh or a nearby table.

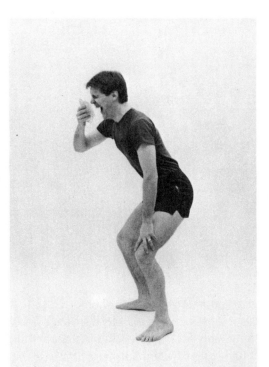

Correct way to sneeze: support the back by placing hand on thigh.

Let me assure you that I do not expect you to be correct in all your actions all the time. Whenever possible, slow down as you perform routine activities to give yourself the time to correct your use. You will undoubtedly have to correct yourself many times a day — it is a normal process everyone goes through. The improved use will gradually replace your old habits.

How long the process takes is different for each person. Some people find that sitting correctly comes easily, but bending correctly is more difficult. For others the opposite may be true. Do not set unrealistic goals for yourself. Realize, instead, that you can now make choices about the way you use your back, and that you are developing a skill that will be immediately beneficial.

APPLICATION TO SPECIFIC MEDICAL PROBLEMS

A variety of medical problems cause back pain, so your first step for dealing with low back pain is to see a physician for a diagnosis. If your physician has determined that your pain is musculoskeletal in origin, the following information will be applicable to your back.

Arched Back (Lordosis)

A back that is habitually arched can damage the structures of the spine in several ways. The delicate spinal facet joints can become irritated because the normal weight borne by the vertebrae falls in the wrong place. Nerve roots become pinched. Back muscles become short and tight, causing them to be easily hurt during activity.

The instructions commonly given for correcting an arched back —tightening the buttock muscles and tucking the pelvis under—only replace one wrong pattern of use with another. Tightening the buttocks is bad for the spine because it prevents free use of the hip joints during walking and bending, and therefore increases strain on the lower back. Tucking under flattens the normal curve in the lower back, keeping the spine from efficient vertical alignment.

The primary muscles for correcting an arched back are the abdominals, not the buttocks, and the instructions for standing (see page 54) also apply to correcting a pronounced arch.

When you stand with your lower back too arched, the front bones of your pelvis (the pubic bones) are dropped too far down.

They should be raised by gently tightening the lower abdominal muscles, which attach all around the front rim of the pelvis. As the muscles start to work, they will correctly balance the pelvis on top of the legs and reduce the arch in the back.

Disc Problems

I am very optimistic about the prognosis for a patient who comes to me with a diagnosis of a herniated, or protruding, disc. Experience has taught me that the body has an amazing ability to deal with this condition. The repair takes place slowly—it may take months—but is successful in most cases.

If you have a history of disc problems (whether or not you have had surgery), you can help keep the problem from recurring by lengthening your entire spine, by using your lower abdominal muscles for support, and by moving freely at your hip joints. An essential part of conservative (non-surgical) treatment is the elimination of all rounding and arching strains from the lower back when you perform your daily activities. Therefore, carefully review the instructions for sitting, standing, bending, and sneezing. Be particularly careful not to slump when sitting for long periods. When you bend to pick something up, be sure to bend from your knees and hips, not from your waist. *Using your abdominal muscles to provide valuable stabilization for your lower back is particularly important if you had surgery a few years ago and are experiencing a recurrence of pain.*

Be careful about which exercises you do. Touching your toes with your knees straight is not good because it places your lower back in the very position that may have caused your disc trouble in the first place. Full sit-ups, from lying down to sitting up all the way, are also hazardous. There are other ways to strengthen the abdominal muscles without endangering the structures of your lower back.

Your physician may prescribe a supporting corset to help keep your spine in correct alignment. But if you depend on the corset to do the entire job, the torso muscles will weaken.

It is possible that you have a condition that requires surgery. Usual indications are unrelenting pain and signs of significant nerve damage, such as muscle weakness or sensory loss. These symptoms are the doctor's clue to carry out further diagnostic procedures.

Chronic Low Back Pain

If you have chronic or frequently recurring low back pain, and a diagnostic workup has ruled out a specific medical problem, the blame probably lies with the way you use your back. Poor use gradually stresses the muscles and ligaments of the lower back until they become so hypersensitive that even simple motions cause pain. In addition to getting treated for the pain, you need to improve your postural habits.

Chronic back pain sufferers have a tendency to respond to emotional stress with muscle tension in the lower back. If this is your pattern, try to become more aware of how your body reacts to what is going on around you and to your own thoughts or emotions. You will be better able to handle demanding situations when you take a few minutes to care for yourself by releasing tense muscles so that your entire torso can lengthen and widen.

Sciatica

The two sciatic nerves (one for each leg) are among the largest nerves in the body. They originate in the lower back, and travel through the deep buttock musculature and down the legs. When irritated they may cause pain, which is called sciatica, and odd sensations along their path such as numbness or tingling. Sciatica has many causes, so if you have pain down one or both legs, you need to see a physician.

The sciatic nerves can be irritated by a protruding disc, the bony spur of an arthritic joint, swollen tissue around a sprained spinal joint, or muscle spasm. In addition, they can be compressed when the buttock muscles are held tight, another reason for my dislike of the frequently prescribed "buttock squeezing" and "tucking under" exercises. Many of my patients have found relief from sciatica when they follow the instructions for walking (see page 56), in which I suggest releasing the buttock muscles with each step forward.

Also effective for an attack of sciatica is to lie on your back with pillows under your knees, so that your legs are completely supported. In this position, the many muscles around the hip joints and in the lower back are encouraged to relax, thus relieving compression and pain. A variation on this position is to lie on the floor and rest your legs on a sofa or chair.

Arthritis

Of the many types of arthritis, osteoarthritis is the kind that most commonly occurs in the spine. Osteoarthritis usually begins around middle age, develops slowly, and seems to be aggravated by the "wear and tear" of daily activities. Particularly helpful for removing mechanical stress from arthritic joints in the lower back are the instructions to lengthen your spine and move freely at the hip joints. People with rheumatoid arthritis, a more serious, systemic illness, report that the Alexander Technique increases their comfort and helps them handle stress more efficiently.

An important concept for those of you with arthritis, no matter what the type or location, is that of *releasing* your muscles (see Chapter 3). Getting rid of unnecessary muscle tension will enable your joints to move more easily and with less pain.

Structural Defects

Perhaps, after looking at your X-rays, your physician has told you that you have *spondylolysis* or *spondylolisthesis*, or *sacralization of a transverse process*. These are three types of bony defects that occasionally occur in the lower part of the spine.

Spondylolysis is a defect or break in the bony ring of a vertebra that allows the front part of the vertebra to slip forward. Spondylolisthesis is the technical term for the slipping forward. The two conditions frequently exist together. If you have the first or both, it is important for you to train your abdominal muscles to protect your lower back during activity. Follow the instructions for standing (page 54), and the abdominal exercises in Chapter 11.

Sacralization of a transverse process (a congenital condition) means that part of a vertebra (the transverse process) is attached to part of the sacrum in a way that does not normally occur. This reduces the normal flexibility of your lower back and can cause pain when you bend to the side. Do not force flexibility, and do not perform any motions that cause pain.

I am including these severe sounding conditions only because I want to ease your fears about them. The main effect they have is to make your back more vulnerable to incorrect use. However, you will respond as well as anyone when you start to improve that use.

6

Shoulder and Upper Back Pain

"The Evolutionary Miracle of the Shoulder Girdle"

BECAUSE OF THE complex and flexible structure of the shoulder girdle, quite a bit can go painfully wrong in this area of the body. Faced with the prospect of having to do something about their shoulders, people usually sigh wearily, picturing hard work ahead. Surprisingly, it is *less* work, not more, that gets the results. As with achieving correct head balance, the solution lies in learning *not to interfere* with the body's beautiful design and built-in balancing mechanisms.

Stand up for a moment and make several large circles with one arm. Notice that you can circle to the front and to the side and that you can reach quite far in back. All this wonderful mobility is an evolutionary gift, the result of skeletal changes that came about as we started to move around on two feet and no longer needed structurally stable arms and shoulders to bear our weight.

We can use our arms for many activities requiring skill, but we can also fall into postural habits that cause our shoulders to be incorrectly balanced, leading to pain in the shoulders, upper back, and arms.

Your first step in learning to use your shoulders correctly is to become more familiar with how this part of your body is structured.

ANATOMY FOR DAILY LIVING

The Bones of the Shoulder Girdle

Start by exploring the structure of your own shoulders. Place the fingertips of your right hand on the front of your chest where the collarbones come close together. Now "walk" your fingers along the left collarbone, all the way out to the left shoulder. At the top of the shoulder you will feel the bumpy area where the collarbone joins the shoulder blade. Now move your hand around to the back of the shoulder and feel the shoulder blade.

Repeat this finger walking using your left hand to feel the right collarbone and right shoulder blade. Then look at the drawings and find these bones on the skeleton.

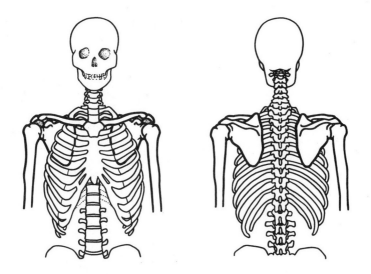

(Left) **Shoulder girdle, front view.** *(Right)* **Shoulder girdle, back view.**

Your two collarbones in front and two shoulder blades in back form a yoke-like structure called the *shoulder girdle*. It is designed to float freely on top of the rib cage. Look again at the drawings and see that the arms do not attach directly to the rib cage, but are hung from this shoulder girdle "yoke."

The Muscles of the Shoulder Girdle

Many muscles connect the shoulder girdle to the head, spine, rib cage, and arms. When the shoulder girdle is continuously off-balance because of poor spinal alignment or unnecessary muscle tension, these muscles may become too stretched or too short. The result can be chronic tension and pain.

As you begin to correct your shoulder girdle balance, the tight, bunched-up muscles will release. As a result, your shoulders will roll forward less, making your neck appear longer.

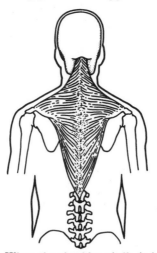

The trapezius muscle: When the shoulder girdle is incorrectly balanced, some areas of this large muscle become too short and others too long.

The most noticeable muscle affected is the *trapezius*, which extends over the neck, shoulders, and upper back. Because it covers such a large area, it is particularly vulnerable to incorrect use. The upper fibers, which attach to the head, neck, and collarbones, often become too short, and the middle and lower fibers, which attach to the shoulder blades and spine, become too stretched.

Many other less visible neck and shoulder muscles are also affected. There may be pain in the muscles themselves, as well as compression of the nerves and blood vessels going into the arms.

You might think that the solution to an incorrectly balanced shoulder girdle would be specific strengthening exercises for some muscles and stretching exercises for others. As with the lower back, however, such an approach would be, at best, only partially effective because our muscles are adaptive creatures, adjusting to the state they are held in most of the time. In other words, an exercise program cannot offset the detrimental effects of many hours spent with faulty spinal alignment and unnecessary muscle tension. Your muscles will gradually adjust for the better as your postural habits improve: overstretched muscles will shorten and give more support, while those that are too tight will lengthen.

The Floating Shoulder Blades

The shoulder blades, which lie against the rib cage in back, are surrounded by muscles. I like to think of them as floating in a sea of muscle because they are so mobile and have no bony attachment to the rib cage. When you make large motions with your arms, the shoulder blades glide around over the back of the rib cage.

LEARNING CORRECT SHOULDER BALANCE

Incorrectly balanced shoulders are usually blamed on delinquent shoulder blade muscles—hence the frequently heard, but ineffective, "hold your shoulders back," with which well-meaning relatives and friends admonish those who are round-shouldered. Frustration and increased upper back pain are the only rewards for those who valiantly attempt to follow this advice. Improving spinal alignment produces much better results. To help you understand why, let me guide you into experiencing both incorrect and correct shoulder balance.

Incorrect Shoulder Balance

Because shoulders are so flexible, their placement is strongly influenced by the structure upon which they rest: the rib cage. The rib cage, in turn, is influenced by spinal alignment.

To see how this relationship works, sit in a chair and slowly go into as much of a slump as you can, noticing how your shoulders passively slip forward. The forward motion occurs because the upper spine and rib cage have become more rounded in back. Remember that the shoulder blades float around in muscle and have no bony attachment to the back of the rib cage to keep them in place.

Now sit up too straight, so that your back arches. This posture, often used in an attempt to correct the slumped one, also prevents the shoulders from balancing correctly because it distorts the spine and rib cage and increases muscle tension.

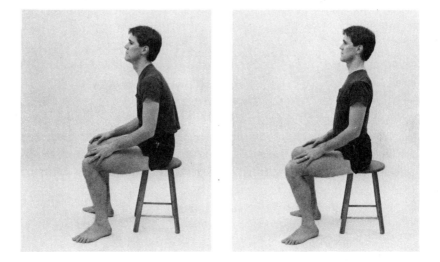

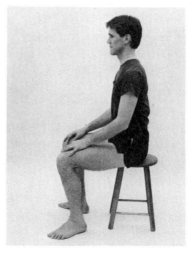

(Top left) **Incorrect: A rounded back interferes with shoulder balance.** *(Top right)* **Incorrect: An arched back also interferes with shoulder balance.** *(Bottom)* **Correct: The shoulders can balance correctly when the torso lengthens and widens.**

Correct Shoulder Balance

To experience correct shoulder balance, forget about shoulder placement, which just creates more tension in the shoulder girdle muscles, and concentrate on spinal alignment. Let me assure you that when your spine is well-aligned and your shoulder muscles are released, your shoulders will automatically balance correctly.

You are going to begin, therefore, by sitting in a chair and applying the first two Concepts of Good Use:

Allow your neck muscles to release so that your head can balance forward and up.

Allow your torso to release into length and width.

As you sit, visualize your head leading your spine up into length. If you are slumping, this image will remind you that you need to correct your sitting alignment. Be sure not to tilt your head back as you lengthen your spine.

Now add the fourth Concept of Good Use:

Allow your shoulders to release out to the sides.

Think of widening across both the front and back of your shoulders. (I also like to think of my spine lengthening up between my shoulder blades as my shoulders release out to the sides.) Do not pull your shoulders back or otherwise try to find a correct position for them, or you will interfere with the dynamic muscular balancing that occurs when your spine lengthens and your shoulder muscles release.

As you think of your shoulders releasing out to the sides, you should feel a lessening of tension in your neck and shoulder muscles. Remember, you are *allowing* your shoulders to release out, not making them do so. Your shoulders will lower slightly if you usually carry them too high. You may also notice that you can breathe more easily because your rib cage is not being compressed in front (which happens when you slump), or in back (which happens when you sit too arched).

It may be difficult for you to accept the fact that simply allowing the shoulders to release, once your torso is lengthening and widening, will result in correct shoulder balance. The reason concepts such as releasing and allowing work so well is that they permit opposing groups of muscles to work together in a coordinated, efficient way. This muscle action occurs on the reflex level and will function well as long as there is no interference from unnecessary muscle tension.

Practicing Correct Shoulder-Arm Use

Because the arms are hung from the bones of the shoulder girdle, the way you use your arms directly affects the way your shoulders are balanced. Learning to use your arms correctly is actually quite simple, and you will be surprised by the feeling of ease you get in your shoulders and upper back.

Pause in your reading for a moment and look at your hands. I want you to become more aware of your hands. As you start to use your arms, you will think of your hands leading the motion and your arms following.

By thinking of your hands leading your arm motion, you can prevent the habit many people have of tensing the shoulders every time they raise their arms. Such unnecessary tension can result in painful neck and shoulder muscles by the end of the day.

To practice using your arms correctly, reach up to touch the top of your head while instructing yourself to let your *hand lead the motion and your arm follow*. Do not expect your shoulder to remain still. It will move along with your arm, particularly when your arm rises above shoulder level. The thought of letting your hand lead and your arm follow allows just the right amount of shoulder motion to occur.

APPLICATION TO DAILY ACTIVITIES

Combing Your Hair

Stand in front of a mirror and watch your head as you raise your arms to comb your hair. Does your head come down to meet your hands? If so, you have lost spinal length and tensed your shoulders and neck muscles unnecessarily.

Pause briefly before raising your arms again so you can *say no to* (inhibit) your impulse to lower your head and tense your shoulders;

think of lengthening up instead. Now start to comb your hair again, this time thinking of bringing your *hands up to your head* instead of your head down to your hands. Notice that you can raise your arms without losing length in your spine and with much less tension in your shoulders. Your shoulders will stay better balanced and you will become more aware of the wonderful flexibility of the shoulders, elbows, and wrists.

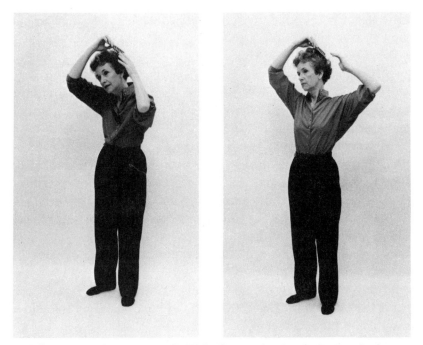

(Left) Incorrect: spine compressed. *(Right)* Correct: head and spine lengthening up.

Reaching Up

Stand and raise one arm as though you were placing an object on a high shelf. Did you feel your back arching and your rib cage moving forward? Arching the back when reaching up is one of the most common causes of shoulder imbalance, and it actually takes strength away from the arms. Our arms get support and power from the large back muscles, and the back needs to be in good alignment—not arched—to give this support. Arching also causes strain and compression in the lower back.

To practice reaching up correctly, stand in profile to a mirror with your arms at your sides. Think of your head leading up and your torso lengthening and widening. Continue this thought as you slowly raise one or both arms in front of you as far as you can comfortably. As your arms start to rise above shoulder level, gently tighten your lower abdominal muscles to keep your back from arching. Raise and lower your arms a few times while checking in the mirror to be sure your back is not arching.

Arching the back when reaching up is an integral part of some activities, such as a tennis serve or certain exercises and dance steps. In such cases, you can arch your back without hurting it by thinking of your entire spine lengthening throughout the movement of reaching and arching. All your torso muscles will then be working to support and protect your spine.

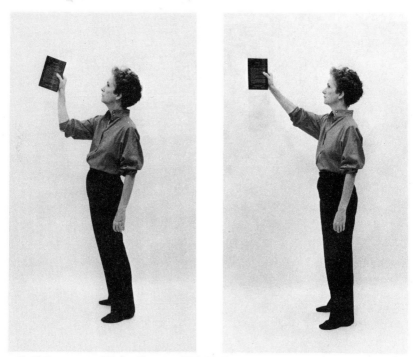

(Left) **Incorrect.** *(Right)* **Correct: Think of your back widening and your lower abdominal muscles gently working as you raise your arm.**

Carrying Heavy Objects

When you carry a heavy object, such as a suitcase, down at your side, there is a damaging downward "drag" on the neck and shoulder muscles. To help your neck and shoulders counteract the weight efficiently, think of an "up energy" going through your entire torso in the direction opposite to the pull of the suitcase.

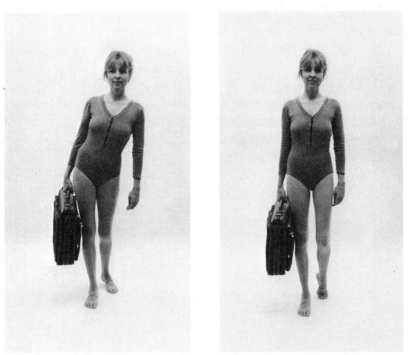

(Left) **Incorrect.** *(Right)* **Correct: Think of your head and torso going up to counteract the downward pull of the suitcase.**

Apply the same "up energy" to your torso when you are carrying a heavy object in front of you. If the object is large and bulky, your torso will automatically lean back to balance the added weight in front. Most people make the mistake of leaning back from the waist, causing strain and compression in the lower back. Think, instead, of your *entire* body leaning slightly back, from your heels all the way up. You will stay in better overall alignment and your shoulder girdle will be more efficiently balanced.

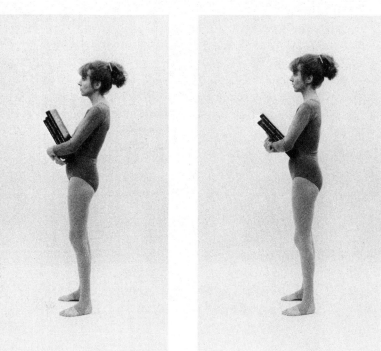

(Left) Incorrect. *(Right)* Correct: Allow your back to stay wide to counterbalance the weight in front.

APPLICATION TO SPECIFIC MEDICAL PROBLEMS

Improved use of the shoulders and upper back is an extremely effective way of alleviating the many musculoskeletal problems that plague this area of the body. Following are some of the more common musculoskeletal conditions and what you can do about them.

Shoulder Tension

The most common cause of shoulder pain is muscle tension. In our complex society it is hard to avoid stressful situations, and the body reacts with increased muscle tension, which eventually becomes so habitual that it does not disappear even when we are relaxing or sleeping.

When you find you are responding to a situation with unnecessary shoulder tension, give yourself a positive alternative:
think of your head leading your spine into length and your shoulders releasing out to the sides. Become aware of your breathing
for a moment; note that you breathe more easily when your shoulder muscles are released. Before going to sleep, and if you wake
during the night, think of releasing your neck and shoulders.
Gradually, the amount of shoulder tension you walk around with
and sleep with will decrease.

Myositis and Trigger Points

The terms *myositis* and *trigger points* refer to forms of chronic
muscle pain. They can occur anywhere in the body, but the upper
back and shoulders are prime targets.

Some physicians use the term myositis, which means inflam-
mation of muscle tissue, to describe chronic, diffuse muscle pain,
and the term trigger points to designate a more localized form of
chronic muscle pain. In either case, the cause (once illness and infec-
tion have been ruled out) is usually the same: prolonged, stressful
use of the muscles because of poor posture and/or emotional tension.

Both myositis and trigger points are usually considered to be the
end result of the following sequence: the muscles are kept in a state
of continual tension . . . which diminishes their blood supply . . .
which deprives them of nutrients and prevents removal of waste
products . . . which results in pain . . . which causes muscle spasm . . .
which causes more pain. The pain-spasm cycle irritates and in-
flames the muscle tissue and interferes with normal muscle
function.

Myositis and trigger points respond well to such treatments as
massage, stretching, and electrical stimulation because all of these
increase the blood supply to the painful muscles. The aim of all of
these treatments is to interrupt the pain-spasm cycle. But unless
you supplement treatment with improving alignment and reducing
muscle tension, the problem can recur. It is also important for
your working setup to be conducive to good use of the body.
Raising your working surface and bringing it closer to you may
help, and a good chair is essential.

Tendinitis and Bursitis

Pain around the shoulder joints can originate from the tendinous attachments of the shoulder muscles, and also from the little cushions (bursae) that lie between the tendon of a muscle and the bone to which that tendon attaches. *Tendinitis* means that a tendon is inflamed, and *bursitis* means that a bursa is inflamed.

Shoulder pain from a tendon or a bursa can be the result of painting your ceiling all day Sunday or spending too many hours typing under the pressure of a deadline. Sudden and prolonged overuse of the shoulders and arms is the immediate cause of the shoulder pain. However, the stage may already have been set for trouble by long-term poor postural habits, which reduce shoulder muscle tolerance for more demanding activity.

Tendinitis or bursitis requires medical treatment, but you can speed the healing process by reducing muscle tension and lengthening your spine so your shoulder girdle can balance correctly.

Round Shoulders

There is a difference between the type of round shoulders that can be immediately corrected by a change in posture because the spine in the upper back is flexible, and the type caused by a more fixed, inflexible curve in that area. The first type is called *functional* and the second, *structural*. Most spines fall somewhere in between.

When your spine is flexible, you can see immediate results in the mirror when you lengthen your torso and release your shoulders out to the sides. It will take thought and patience to correct your round-shouldered posture, but it is important because the condition can gradually become more permanent (structural).

For a structurally (less flexible) rounded upper back, some correction is usually possible. You can also help prevent the condition from becoming worse. Many people believe that a rounded upper back and shoulders will always get more rounded as time passes, but I strongly disagree. The main factor in determining whether or not you become more round shouldered is how you *use* your back.

Some occupations tend to encourage a round-shouldered posture. I have been consulted by a number of young dentists who were concerned because of the posture their work requires. I have three suggestions to give them and others whose work may lead to a rounded upper back: (1) try to change your working position to minimize the need to bend forward; (2) bend forward with as much length in the spine as possible (instead of "telescoping" the spine by relaxing into a slump); and (3) practice "antidote movements" frequently throughout the working day—simple arm and upper back stretches to take the body into new positions. These stretches will feel good because they relieve joint pressure and muscle fatigue; more important, they help prevent the upper back from gradually becoming fixed in a rounded position.

Tutors, counselors, psychologists, and others who work with people on a one-to-one basis also need to watch how they use their upper back. I have been told by many in these professions that they constantly catch themselves leaning forward toward their clients in a way that takes the head, neck, and shoulders out of good alignment, and that they feel the resultant strain at the end of the day. Those I have taught find they can make postural changes (sometimes a change in seating arrangement helps) without losing the important personal connection they want to have with their clients. In other words, it is not necessary to sacrifice your neck, shoulders and upper back in order to do such work effectively.

A rounded upper back can sometimes be painful, and then it becomes a serious problem. Writers, musicians, and computer programmers are all fair game. One writer came to me with such severe upper back and arm pain that she could not use her typewriter. Her physician had determined that the pain was directly related to poor body positioning and very tense muscles while working, and I, too, could see that the postural habits of many years were responsible. In addition to teaching her how to work with a more lengthened spine and released shoulders, I made sure she had a chair that could be pulled up close to the typing table and gave good support to her lower back (see Chapter 7, "Buying a Good Desk Chair"). The height of the working surface is also important. If it is too high, it can cause unnecessary shoulder and arm tension; if too low, it can cause slumping. We adjusted the height of the typewriter so her elbows could be bent approximately 90 degrees, and she had her eyeglasses prescription changed so she could read at the proper distance for working with her spine lengthened. As her use of her back improved, the pain disappeared, and she is now able to work for many hours without discomfort.

I would like to point out that even if the appearance of your upper back is more structurally curved then you are happy with, you are probably appraising yourself more critically than others do. Moreover, when you look in the mirror your eyes most likely focus on whatever part of yourself you do not like, whereas others look at you and see your entire self. A large part of the impression we make on others is determined by the way we use the energy in our bodies. Therefore, if your entire torso has an "up energy," and if you are letting your head lead your spine into length, other people will not notice whether your upper back is more or less rounded.

Ankylosing Spondylitis

A few years ago a man in his middle fifties with a moderate curve in his upper back but excellent overall posture came to me for Alexander lessons. He had no particular musculoskeletal complaint, just a general interest in the Alexander Technique.

When I examined his back I found his spine to be completely rigid, a condition unusual for someone of his age. In response to questions regarding his medical history, he said that twenty years ago he had been diagnosed as having *ankylosing spondylitis*, an arthritic condition in which the spine gradually loses its flexibility and becomes rigid. He told me that because he is a fighter by nature, he had said to himself that if his spine was going to become rigid, at least it could do so in a "good posture" alignment. Most people with ankylosing spondylitis become more and more curved forward in the head, neck, and upper back. He had been able to avoid this by exercising regularly and being very diligent about his sitting and standing alignment.

If you have ankylosing spondylitis, you should be especially aware of your postural habits, eliminating as much as possible any tendency to slump forward when sitting or bending down. When you sleep, try to keep your back as straight as you can by not curling up. You should also consult a physical therapist for appropriate exercises to keep your back and rib cage as limber as possible.

7

Positions We All Get Into

A few years ago, a new patient phoned me with a strange complaint: he could not fit into his car. What led to his predicament? Being very tall but an habitual slumper, he had bought a car that fit his slumped stature. During his first Alexander lesson the man's spine achieved its true length, which he maintained as he walked to his car. Once inside the car, he found his head pressed against the roof! He said he had to choose between raising the roof and telescoping his spine, but he knew what my response would be—to get another car with more head room.

AS YOU BECOME more aware of how to use your back correctly, you will discover how your physical surroundings can sometimes stand in your way. In addition to cars with insufficient head room, there are desk chairs that give status but no back support, and low bathroom sinks that force you to sacrifice your spine for the sake of clean teeth. In most cases, there are ways to win the battle against unfriendly furnishings.

SLEEPING

All my back patients ask what positions they should sleep in. Lying on your side or back is the safest if you have back pain. The question of using or nor using a pillow depends on your position. In general, I am a strong believer in letting pillows help support the body. Even though they may get displaced during the night, they will at least help for a while, and you will gradually be able to keep them in position for longer periods of time. Foam pillows, however, do not stay where they are put.

Sleeping on Your Side

Choose a firm, fairly thick pillow for under your head and neck. It will prevent your head from dropping down toward the mattress and it will take some pressure off the shoulder you are lying on. To increase your comfort further, particularly if you have lower back pain, place a pillow between your knees to prevent pull on your lower back.

If your problem area is the neck or shoulders, place a small pillow in front of you to support the arm that is uppermost. The pillow will prevent that arm and shoulder from dropping forward toward the mattress and pulling on your neck and upper back.

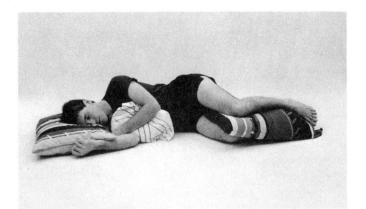

Sleeping on Your Back

Place a pillow under your head (the size depends on comfort) and one or more large pillows under your knees.

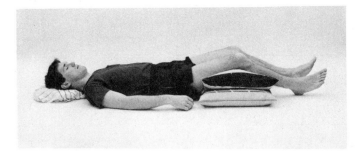

Sleeping on Your Stomach

You should probably avoid this position. However, if you can't get to sleep any other way, place a pillow under your stomach to prevent your back from arching. Do not put a pillow under your head because it will tilt your head back and compress your neck.

An excellent variation on stomach sleeping is to bend one leg up to the side so that you are slightly raised on that side. Now place a pillow partially under your stomach and chest to support the part of you that is raised.

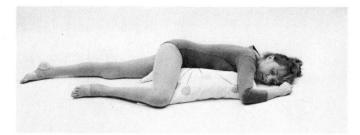

What About the Mattress?

A firm mattress is preferable because it keeps the head, neck, and torso in good alignment. A mattress that is too soft allows the body to sag in various places, causing strain on muscles, ligaments, and joints. Some people find a very firm mattress uncomfortable but they buy it anyway, thinking it will solve their back problems. It is better to select the firmest one upon which you can sleep comfortably.

Waterbeds

Some people with back problems find a waterbed wonderful; others hurt more after using one. Your best guide is how your back feels in the morning. Just be sure not to fill it so full that it becomes uncomfortably hard. The bed should give good overall support (so you do not sag out of alignment) but still conform gently to the curves of your body.

READING IN BED

Being addicted to this wonderful activity myself, I have found ways of reading in bed that do not endanger my back. The trick is to either lie down so that your back is flat against the mattress, or sit all the way up with good back support. In either case, the knees should be bent and you should use pillows for support.

Lying on Your Back

Even though the following arrangement requires four or five pillows, it is well worth the effort if reading in bed happens to be one of your pleasures in life. Place a pillow under your head so that you are raised up just enough for reading. Place a pillow under each elbow to raise your arms slightly. Bend your knees up and place a pillow under the covers to prop your feet against, so they do not slide down. Now rest the book against your thighs. If the book is too far away, place a small pillow behind it. This position is very relaxing and will not hurt your back or your neck.

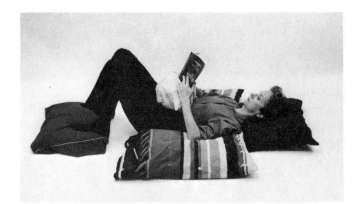

Sitting

Place two standard bed pillows behind your back, pushing the one closest to you down into the small of your back to give your lower back extra support. Place another pillow under your knees. A small pillow under the book will mean you do not have to hold it up with your arms.

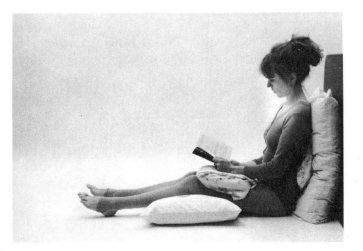

Lying on Your Side

This position can be comfortable for short periods. Use a large pillow under your head and neck (or you can put two standard pillows into one pillow case). Prop the book against another pillow so that it is at a good angle for reading.

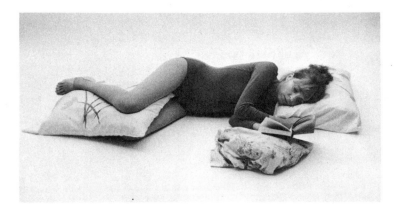

SEXUAL ACTIVITY

Many people with low back pain are apprehensive about having sexual relations because they are afraid of hurting their back and causing more pain.

My advice to my patients is that sexual activity need not be avoided so long as safe and pain-free positions can be found. Actually, many people find the pelvic motions beneficial for the back. The feeling of well-being that comes from a satisfying sexual experience benefits you physically as well as emotionally, and therefore will actually increase your body's recuperative powers.

Sexual intercourse should be avoided if you have acute back pain and muscle spasm because the activity may trigger more muscle spasm. If you are able to work and carry out other normal activities, however, you need not avoid sex. Just be sure your partner understands the need to give special attention to positions because of your back condition.

A good general guideline for protecting your back during sexual intercourse is to have your hips and knees bent. The drawings illustrate two positions safe for both of you. Notice how the man can be on his hands and knees when in the superior position if his partner is raised up on pillows.

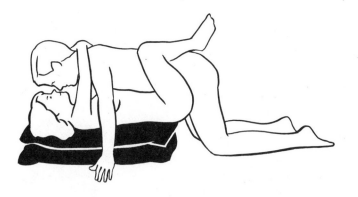

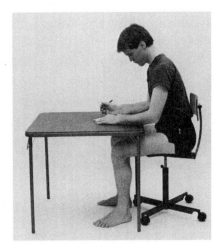

Lying "spoon fashion" is also safe for your back: you both lie on your side with the woman's back to the man's front.

Be adventurous in finding positions comfortable and good for you both. Try to remember that your back will do better if it is not too arched, too rounded, or twisted. Also, be sure your partner does not inadvertently force your knees too close to your chest if this puts an uncomfortable strain on your lower back.

SITTING AT YOUR DESK

There are two ways to sit at a desk without hurting your back:

1. Keep your back lengthened and lean forward from your hip joints. Sitting this way is good for the back, but it becomes tiring after a while. It should be alternated with the second method.

2. Pull your chair very close to the desk so the back of the chair can support your back. If the chair cannot be pulled close enough, or the seat is too deep for you, place a pillow behind you for better support.

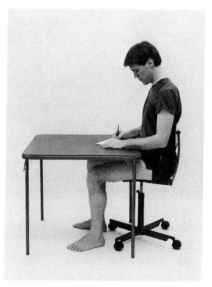

No matter how hard you may try, sitting correctly at your desk for long periods of time is almost impossible if you do not have a good chair.

How to Buy a Good Desk Chair

The following guidelines will help you purchase a desk chair that protects your back by encouraging you to sit correctly:

1. Your chair must give your lower back enough support to discourage slumping. Therefore, the back of the chair should curve forward slightly toward your lower back. Most secretarial-type chairs (without arms) give good support; most executive-type chairs do not.

2. You must be able to pull the chair up close to the desk. If the chair has arms, they must be low enough to fit under the desk.

3. Your feet should rest comfortably on the floor when you are sitting all the way back in the seat.

4. The chair seat should give firm support even if it is upholstered.

5. A good feature of some desk chairs is an adjustable seat and back. Check that the back can be locked in place. Do not buy a chair that has a back that gives way when you lean against it. These have a flexible or spring-loaded bar connecting the back to the seat.

Using a Kneeling Chair

Kneeling chairs provide a different way of sitting. This innovative seat encourages good spinal alignment because it permits the pelvis to balance correctly (sit-bones pointing down) and has no back to slump against. You can choose from several different models: some are on wheels, some rock, and some adjust in height.

Do not rush into buying one, however, until you give it a lengthy try in the store. Many people find these chairs very comfortable; others cannot tolerate the pressure on the knees and shins for very long. I use mine for brief periods as an alternative to my regular desk chair.

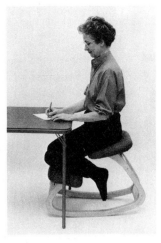

TALKING ON THE PHONE

Telephones bring out our worst in terms of body use. They make it almost impossible not to slump, twist, and scrunch.

To help your spine stay lengthened and your shoulders better balanced when holding the phone to your ear, support your arm in a raised position by resting your elbow on a pile of books or small card file. If you can't count on having something handy, get a bean bag for this purpose.

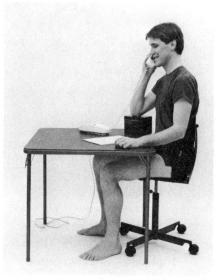

If you frequently prop the phone between your head and shoulders when you talk, I strongly recommend that you get a telephone headset to replace the standard hand-held part of your phone. This habit is so ruinous to the body that I would like to see all phones equipped with headsets. They are lightweight and comfortable and, more important, they allow you to keep your head, neck, and shoulders in good alignment. Headsets are for sale at most stores that specialize in telephones and telephone accessories.

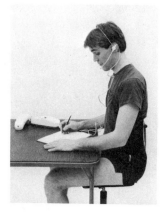

READING IN A CHAIR

The temptation when sitting and reading (or sewing, knitting, etc.) is to slump down to your book because holding it up tires your arms. The solution is quite simple: sit all the way back in the seat and put a pillow in your lap under the book. You will be surprised how comfortable this is. If the chair is too deep, place another pillow behind you.

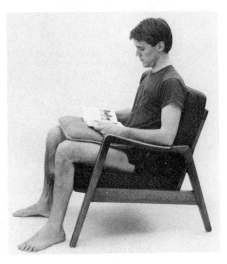

SHAVING OR PUTTING ON MAKE-UP

The awkward position of leaning forward over the sink to see yourself in the mirror while shaving or putting on make-up is extremely hard on the back, neck, and shoulders. As with teeth brushing (see below), placing one foot on the toilet, tub rim, or stool will take strain off your back. A better option would be to get a mirror that can be pulled toward you.

BRUSHING YOUR TEETH

Bending over the bathroom sink without hurting your back is one of modern life's more formidable challenges. You need to bend with your knees and hip joints while keeping your spine lengthened. If the layout of your bathroom permits, place one foot on top of the toilet or rim of the tub while bending forward. Or use a low step stool or box that you keep by the sink. When neither of these is possible, take a wide stance, bend both your knees, and lean forward from your hip joints while lengthening your back. Try to keep one hand free to place on the sink for support.

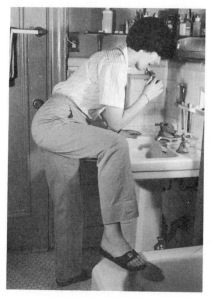

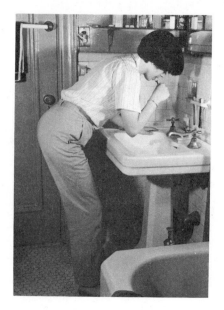

TRAVELING BY PLANE, TRAIN, OR BUS

The first thing I do after getting on a plane is to find two pillows; I recommend you do the same. Place one pillow in the small of your back and the other on your lap under your book or magazine. If you think that pillows will not be supplied, take along a sweater or compressible jacket to support your lower back. If possible, get up and walk around briefly every hour to prevent your back from becoming stiff and fatigued.

DRIVING

In addition to the need for sufficient head room, good support for the lower back is essential when you are driving. A firm, wedge-shaped back rest, or combination back and seat support, can usually be purchased where car accessories are sold. Most wedge-shaped back supports come with instructions to put the thinner edge on top. I advise my patients to do the reverse. Placing the thicker edge on top keeps your entire torso more vertical.

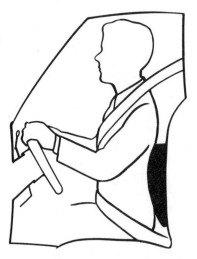

Try to avoid cars with seats that slant way back because they force you to round your upper back and hold your head and neck too far forward. If you drive regularly in this poor alignment, you may develop serious neck and upper back pain. You should have sufficient back support to keep your torso almost vertical and to support your lower back so that you do not slump.

MEDITATING

More and more people spend time each day in some form of meditation. Unfortunately, many of them have developed distracting back pain.

The most common position used for meditation, and the one that causes most back discomfort, is sitting cross-legged on the floor. Very few people have enough flexibility in their hip joints and legs to sit this way without going into a slumped posture. There is an easy solution: place a firm cushion under your hips but *not* under your legs. You will notice that without the cushion, your lower back is forced to become rounded, but with the cushion, you are able to keep your head, neck, and torso in good vertical alignment.

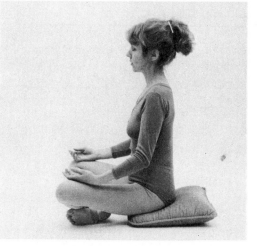

Whether you sit in a chair or on the floor, always consider your body when you meditate. When you position yourself correctly, so that your spine can lengthen and all your torso muscles balance efficiently, the time you spend meditating will also serve as valuable healing time for your back.

Be inventive about modifying your physical surroundings to encourage good use of your back. If necessary, get more pillows for the bedroom and throw pillows for the living room couch. When buying new dining room or kitchen chairs, select a style that gives good back support. Also do not hesitate to request—politely but firmly—that you be given a chair at work that supports your back properly.

8

Breathing Correctly To Ease Back Pain

HAS TENSION AND SPASM in your back muscles ever interfered with your breathing? It may not have occurred to you that by improving your breathing you could have reduced the pain.

Most people do not give breathing much thought except to be glad they are doing it. And yet, how we breathe affects every part of the body, including the back muscles. Take a moment to place both hands on your rib cage in back and feel your breathing cycle. Now lower your hands slightly to about waist level; you will again feel yourself breathe, though less noticeably. All the back muscles, whether they lie on the ribs or below them, are influenced by our breathing and, conversely, our breathing is influenced by the back muscles.

Emotional stress, as well as poor postural habits, can interfere with our breathing patterns. Even after the stress has been dealt with and eliminated, breathing sometimes remains inefficient simply out of habit. By practicing good breathing, you will be able to change these habits.

WHAT IS GOOD BREATHING?

Correct breathing is characterized by an easeful in-and-out motion of the rib cage and free use of the diaphragm, the main breathing muscle. It should feel effortless.

The diaphragm is attached all around to the lower ribs and to some vertebrae in back. I want you to visualize it as a dome-shaped floor of the rib cage. When you breathe in, the dome lowers and the lower ribs flare out slightly to the sides. The front and back walls of the rib cage also move away from each other. These small changes make more space for air to flow in; the opposite must happen for the used air to leave the body. Breathing out is largely passive due to the elasticity of the lungs and chest wall, and requires no noticeable muscle effort unless you are coughing, sneezing, or exercising vigorously.

Many people think that blowing up the chest like a balloon indicates good breathing. Actually, using this image as a guide ignores the fact that breathing out is as important as breathing in. It also creates tension throughout the body. Others believe they can breathe more deeply by sucking in their abdominal muscles. What actually happens, though, is that deep breathing is prevented because the tight abdominal muscles interfere with the lowering of the diaphragm. Still others use the upper chest and neck muscles too much and make minimal use of the diaphragm, causing a shallow breathing pattern. Quiet, normal breathing should be done mainly with the diaphragm and lower ribs.

You do not have to force yourself to breathe because your body does this automatically based on how much oxygen you need. When you are very active you breathe more quickly and your rib cage moves more than when you are less active.

Here are two breathing concepts you can practice anytime, whether you are lying down, sitting, or being more active. Both emphasize the idea of *doing less* to improve your breathing.

Think of releasing all the muscles surrounding your torso to allow breathing to occur.

Your rib cage is cylindrical in shape and should move in and out in all directions (with motion more noticeable in the lower ribs).

Think of allowing air to flow into and out of your lungs, rather than pulling it in or pushing it out.

When your diaphragm lowers and your ribs move out in all directions, a partial vacuum is created inside your rib cage that helps the outside air flow into the lungs, making it unnecessary to pull the air in. When the expansion of the rib cage reverses itself, the air is expelled without conscious effort.

A BREATHING EXERCISE TO REDUCE BACK SPASM

Muscle spasm is often prolonged due to a pain-tension cycle—pain causes more tension, which then causes more pain, until eventually the back muscles become locked in spasm. The following exercise, which I prefer to call a "breathing experience" so you do not think of it as requiring vigorous breathing, can help you end this cycle. It can be as effective (or in some cases more so) as procaine injections, given for the same purpose.

Lie on your back—on the floor or in bed, whichever is more comfortable—with a small pillow under your head and a large one under your knees. Let your legs relax on the pillow. Close your eyes and visualize your rib cage as an empty cylinder, and give the cylinder a flexible floor (the diaphragm muscle). Imagine yourself as a tiny speck of consciousness floating in the center of the cylinder. As you breathe in, watch the walls and floor gently move away from you, and as you breathe out, watch them gently move toward you.

Hold onto this image for a few moments. You will begin to be aware of the gentle in-and-out motion of your rib cage. If you place a hand just below your ribs in front, you will feel a slight rise (when you breathe in) and fall (when you breathe out) of your body that lets you know that the diaphragm is working freely.

The gentle rib cage and diaphragm motion has the effect of giving your back a soothing massage from the *inside* of your body. Gradually your entire body and mind will relax and give your back muscles a chance to get out of spasm. If you practice every day for a few weeks — not just when your back is in spasm — your body will gradually become accustomed to a more beneficial breathing pattern.

9

Emergency Treatment for the Back About To Go into Spasm

"I can't always tell <u>what</u> causes my back to get into trouble, but I usually know <u>when</u> it is about to give me a hard time."

"My back gives me warning signals by feeling tight a few days before it goes into spasm."

ALTHOUGH NOT EVERYONE'S back sends out a warning, I hear such comments fairly often, and they are usually coupled with the statement, "I wish there were something I could do besides just feeling helpless as my back proceeds to get worse."

In this chapter I am going to teach you what you *can* do under these circumstances. The following mind-body sequence of movements is an effective way of staving off muscle spasm in the back. I like to think of it as a form of "body meditation."

Read through the instructions a few times before starting to practice. Pay particular attention to the mental instructions. They will be familiar because they are based on Alexander's Concepts of Good Use.

Step 1: Lengthen Head and Torso Up

Stand with your feet a few inches apart. Think of releasing your neck muscles so that your head can ease up off your neck. Add the thought to let your torso lengthen and widen and follow your head up.

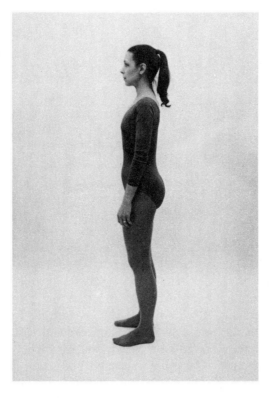

Step 2: Bend into a Squat

Think of releasing your knees forward and away from each other as you bend down into a squat. As you go down, lean forward from your hip joints and reach out with your hands toward the floor in front. You may touch the floor with your fingertips for balance. Let your heels come off the floor as you go down, and think of your head leading your spine into length.

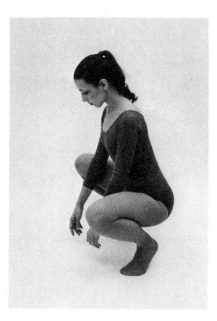

Step 3: Go onto Hands and Knees

From the squatting position go onto your hands and knees.
Stay there for a few moments while you think of lengthening
out through the top of your head. You should be looking down
at the floor so the back of your neck can lengthen.

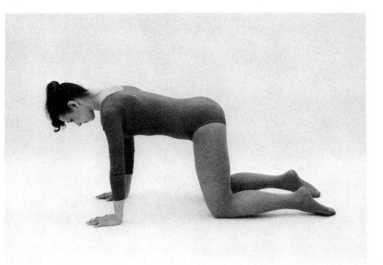

Step 4: Crawl Forward and Back

Slowly crawl forward 6 steps and then backwards 6 steps (each knee moving forward or backwards is 1 step). Use any sequence of hand-knee action that comes naturally to you. As you crawl, be aware of the gentle motion that occurs throughout your spine and pelvis. The motion will help reduce or help prevent muscle spasm.

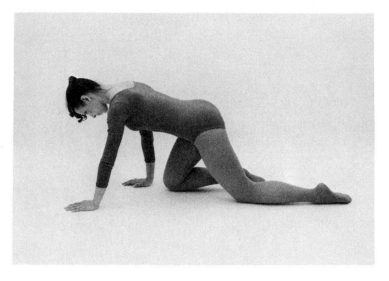

Step 5: Fold-Up

Slowly move your torso back toward your heels and go into the "fold-up" position with your head and arms resting on the floor in front of you. If your lower back is tight you may not be able to fold completely (tightness in your knees may also limit you). Go only as far as you can comfortably. Stay in this position while you breathe in and out 5 times in a relaxed way.

Getting into this position when your back is askew due to muscle spasm will help return your pelvis and spine to correct alignment. It will also help whenever your back feels tired or tight.

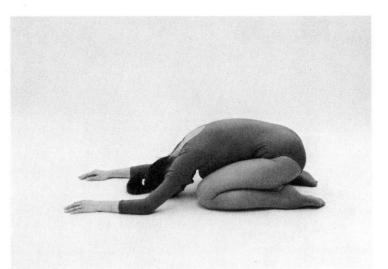

Step 6: Do Knee Circles

Roll slowly onto your back, bring both knees up toward your chest, and place a hand on each knee. Slowly move both knees in small circles (so that they separate and come together again), 5 times in one direction and 5 times in the other. Think of your head leading your spine into length when your knees come close to your chest. As your knees circle, you will feel your pelvis gently rocking. The motion will reduce tension and spasm in your lower back.

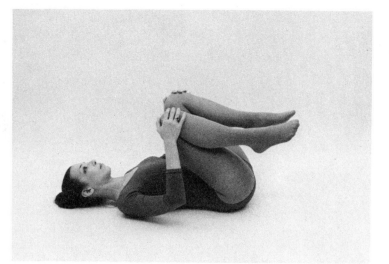

Step 7: Review the Concepts of Good Use

Remain on your back and place your feet on the floor
(knees bent). Rest in this position while mentally reviewing
Alexander's Concepts of Good Use. This will help the Concepts carry over when you get up and move around.

*Allow your neck muscles to release so your head is not pulled
into your neck.*

*Allow your torso to release into length and width, and
lengthen toward your head.*

Allow your legs to release away from your pelvis.

Allow your shoulders to release out to the sides.

Now think of releasing all the muscles around your torso
to allow your ribs to move freely in and out as you breathe.

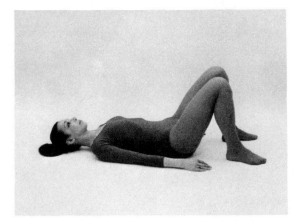

Step 8: Return to Hands and Knees

Slowly roll over onto your hands and knees and stay there a moment while thinking of your back releasing into length.

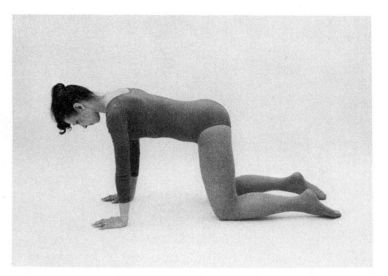

Step 9: Return to Fold-Up Position

Slowly move your torso into the fold-up position and stay there for a moment. It may seem easier this time. Return to your hands and knees.

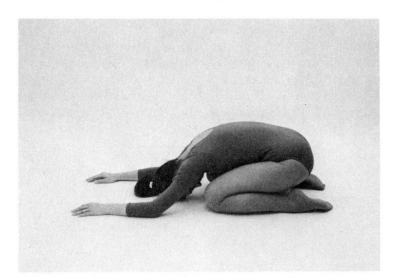

Step 10: Return to Squatting

Change the position of your feet so that your toes are tucked under (bottom of toes touching floor), and move your knees apart. Place your hands on the floor in front of you to help push your hips back over your feet until you are in a squat.

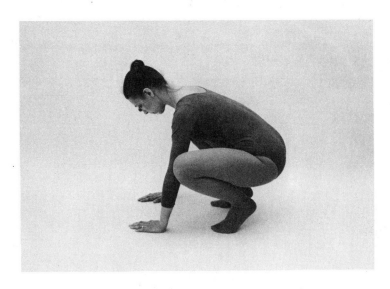

Step 11: Return to Standing

Slowly stand up, getting yourself started by pushing off the
floor with your hands. Think of your head leading your spine
into length.

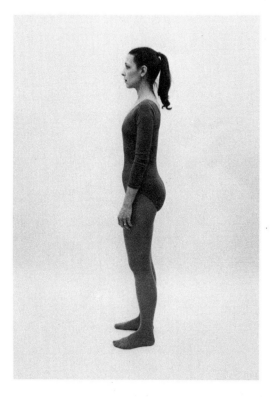

Step 12: Walk

Walk around while thinking of your head and spine lengthening up and your legs moving forward freely from your hip joints.

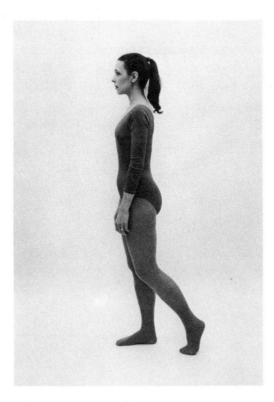

Take as much time as you like for the entire movement sequence. The only rule is not to do it quickly. If one of the positions feels particularly comfortable for your back, remain in it for awhile before going on to the next step.

Some of the steps can be helpful used alone. Try the fold-up position and the knee circles whenever your back feels tired or tight. If you happen to be in the middle of a public place and you start feeling a tightness or pressure across the lower back (perhaps after standing or walking for a long time), you won't be able to lie down, but you can get into the squatting position for a moment, which will ease the pressure. Or you can alternately raise your knees up toward your chest while standing, which will also help your lower back feel better.

Since your mind and body are working together during this movement sequence, it has an "unstressing" effect similar to that of meditation. I therefore recommend that you repeat it daily as a preventive measure, even when your back is not sending out warning signals.

10

What About Supportive Collars and Corsets?

ORTHOPEDIC COLLARS FOR the neck and corsets for the back serve two main purposes. They give support and they minimize spinal motions that may interfere with healing. These are worthy functions and well justify the use of such devices. However, their beneficial effects can be sabotaged by improper fit and insufficient instructions to the patient for their use. Following are some guidelines for deriving the most benefit from the collar or back support that may have been prescribed for you.

SUPPORTIVE COLLARS

Whenever I see someone on the street wearing a neck collar that is higher in front than in back, I have the urge to rush up to that person and turn the collar around. Most of the time my impulse would be correct; occasionally it would be wrong. Let me explain what factors would make the difference, to help you determine whether you are wearing your collar correctly.

Many of the more common neck problems are caused or aggravated by habitually pulling the head back and down, which compresses the neck. If you are wearing a supportive collar that is higher in front than in back, it is forcing your chin up and the back of your head down on your neck. Your collar is actually reinforcing the postural habit that most likely caused your neck problem in the first place.

Some types of soft neck collars that fasten with Velcro are prime offenders because they are narrow at the ends, which most people put in back, and wider in the middle. These collars serve you better if you simply turn them around so that they fasten in front. In this position, the collar can do its supporting job and at the same time remind you not to walk around with your head pulled back and down. Also, when your collar is lower in front, you can look down by simply tilting your head forward instead of straining your neck and shoulders.

There are other, well-designed, collars that fasten with Velcro in back. They have a built-in depression in front for the chin and therefore do not force your head back and down. They come in different sizes so you can be fitted for the correct width under your chin.

In some instances it is appropriate for a supportive collar to keep the head tilted slightly back. If, for example, you have had a neck injury that has overstretched the ligaments in the back of your neck, they may need to be kept shortened while they heal. Your physician or physical therapist will determine whether your head needs to be held in this position.

A comfortable way to give your neck support while you sleep is to make a "towel collar." Spread out a standard size bath towel and roll it up lengthwise into a long, thin roll. Place the center of the rolled-up towel under your chin, cross the ends in back, and drape the ends forward over your shoulders. Now pull the front of the towel down slightly so that it makes a comfortable chin rest. You can hold the ends in place with masking tape.

If the physician who prescribed your collar tells you that you no longer need to wear it continuously, try to wean yourself of its support by removing it for longer periods each day. Until you are completely free of the collar, it is a good idea to continue wearing it when you are in a moving vehicle, which is subject to sudden jolting motions.

SUPPORTIVE CORSETS

"When I no longer need this monster I'll use it as a planter," said a patient who had worn a back support for twenty years. I am happy to say that this unique use of an orthopedic corset did come to pass once the patient learned to do for herself what the corset had been doing for her all those years.

There are, of course, exceptional circumstances in which a back support needs to be worn on a permanent basis. For the most part, however, a supportive corset should be used as a temporary aid to recovery and then put in the closet, to be used again only if severe symptoms recur and the corset helped previously.

The purpose of the corset is to support the back and help maintain correct spinal alignment during activity. A corset should make your back feel better, it should remind you to use your back correctly, and it should allow you to be more active with less fatigue in your back muscles. If you have been confined to your bed because of back pain, you may find it helpful to wear a corset during your first week on your feet. You may also benefit from wearing one for the next few weeks for activities known to be hard on the back, such as standing for a long time or traveling.

Although a corset can be helpful at times, many people have told me that their backs do just as well, or better, without one. Medical opinion is divided. Given the same ailing back, one physician will prescribe a corset; another will not.

If you are presently wearing a corset, have confidence in your ability to determine whether or not it is helping your back. "Listen" to the way your back responds. The corset may help you feel more secure and less tired, and therefore able to return to your normal activities sooner. Or you may find the restrictiveness and pressure of the corset such an irritant that you and your back become more tense. In that case, discuss these reactions with your physician, who will decide if your back still needs the added stability of the corset.

Despite differences of opinion regarding short-term use, most experts agree that dependency on a supportive corset should be avoided. If you have become dependent on a corset, you may need to wean yourself from it gradually. Discuss this with your doctor.

Be sure to follow the instructions for maintaining spinal length when sitting and bending. Sit in firm chairs, avoid carrying heavy packages, and lie down as often as necessary to avoid fatigue.

TYPES OF CORSETS

One type of corset is relatively narrow and is used specifically for sacroiliac joint instability. It is worn tightly around the pelvis. Although the purpose of this belt-like corset is to help the sacroiliac joints gradually gain stability, it will be waging a losing battle if you continually sit in a slump and bend forward from the waist—two harmful habits that put stress on the sacroiliac joints. Habitually sitting with your pelvis askew, rather than placing your hips squarely in the chair, will also undermine the sacroiliac joints. In other words, using a sacroiliac support is a waste of time unless you are also using your back correctly.

There are different types of flexible corsets, ranging from those with plastic stays or a firm pad in back, to the more supportive type with metal bars that need to be custom shaped to each wearer. Which one you need depends on how much spinal motion should be restricted and how much of the spine needs support.

It is important to realize that flexible corsets limit spinal motion but do not prevent it. Experiment while wearing yours to see how much you can change your spinal alignment. With any type of corset that is not completely rigid, part of the job of aligning your spine correctly remains with you—a desirable attribute in a corset, in my opinion.

A completely rigid support, referred to as a back "brace," should be avoided unless absolutely necessary. This type undermines the strength of the abdominal and back muscles because the wearer tends to lean against it for support, instead of using the muscles to hold up the body. Fortunately, such a restrictive brace is seldom prescribed for back pain these days.

It is far better to use the abdominal muscles (your natural corset) efficiently than any store-bought corset. Your own muscles can reduce the forward and downward pull of the abdominal area on the lower back and help maintain good spinal alignment. Remember, the more you use your corset, the sooner it wears out; the more you use your abdominal muscles, the stronger they get.

11

Healing Exercises for the Back

TO MOVE IS TO BE ALIVE, and to stretch and strengthen the body is to enhance the experience of living. Those who exercise for enjoyment already agree with this sentiment; those with disabling back pain often view exercising with apprehension.

If you have never looked upon exercising with an enthusiastic eye, I hope to change your attitude by making you more knowledgeable about what you are doing when you exercise, why you are doing it, and how to do it in the best possible way.

Let me reiterate, however, that because back pain can be a symptom of a variety of ailments, you should not start an exercise program without first consulting a physician.

WHY IS EXERCISING NECESSARY?

If you were to carry a skeleton to the center of a room and expect it to stand there all by itself, you would be disappointed. Without muscles to keep it upright, it would soon be a pile of bones on the floor. Your muscles will carry out their supportive function better when a daily exercise program keeps them strong and flexible.

Your skeleton itself, particularly the spine, must also be considered. The spine is an intricately jointed structure that loses its flexibility, and therefore its well-being, when it is not moved regularly in all directions.

You may be tempted to stop exercising as soon as your back feels better. "I stopped doing my exercises," is the explanation I hear from patients who didn't realize how quickly their muscles would lose tone and their spine flexibility, leading to a recurrence of pain. Develop the self-discipline to keep up your exercise routine even when it has already helped you recover. A good exercise program is not only curative but protective, and will help prevent further problems from developing.

THE BEST WAY TO EXERCISE

How you do your exercises is as important as which ones you do, and the how concerns your mind as well as your body. Use your exercise time to "center" yourself both mentally and physically. When you exercise, your body should not be in one part of the universe while your mind is in another. Focusing your thoughts on the flow of movement will encourage your mind and body to work harmoniously. Never rush through your exercises. If you do not have the time to go through all the recommended repetitions carefully, do fewer—but do them correctly.

While you exercise it is important to avoid faulty postural habits, such as pulling the head back and down and compressing the spine, or the exercises themselves will reinforce these habits. You should, therefore, be thinking of the Concepts of Good Use as you exercise. Spinal lengthening is particularly important. When you remember to lengthen your spine, you protect the structures of your back because lengthening allows all the muscles that spiral around your torso to give good support.

With stretching exercises, think of *releasing* into the stretch rather than using force. As an example: when you are stretching the hamstring muscles (in the back of the thighs), do not use a bouncing motion, but imagine the muscles releasing and elongating as you apply a steady, gentle pull for 20 seconds. Ease up on the pull and then repeat three or four times. Painful stretching is not as productive as gentle persuasion. Any time the stretch produces pain, you are actually working against yourself because the body's response is to tighten up even more.

HOW TO SELECT BENEFICIAL EXERCISES

If your back pain is severe enough for you to seek medical help, your exercise program will probably be tailored to your particular back by your physician, a physical therapist, or an exercise specialist. However, if your physician feels you do not need to be under his or her care, the following guidelines will help you make up your own program.

1. You should not do exercises that are, in themselves, harmful. There are two that I believe fall in this category:

> *Toe touching* while standing with the knees straight is harmful for most people because it puts a strain on the lower back. The exception is for those whose hamstrings are *already* so limber that they can keep their knees straight and touch their toes with ease.
> *Head rolls* done with the neck muscles completely relaxed cause the delicate joint surfaces in the neck to be ground together. Therefore, always keep some supportive tone in your neck as you circle your head by thinking of your head easing up off your neck.

2. You need a balanced variety of exercises so that as you strengthen one set of muscles (such as the abdominals), you also spend time working their opposite set (the back muscles).

3. An important and yet seldom recognized criterion is to avoid any exercise that reinforces poor postural habits. If, for example, your back is too arched, you should not do exercises that require you to arch your back until you have corrected this

postural pattern. Or, if you sit most of the day and tend to slump, you should not do full sit-ups (from lying down to sitting all the way up) because they will reinforce your tendency to be round-shouldered. (To understand how this exercise forces the body into poor alignment, stop in the middle of a sit-up and observe how your head, neck, shoulders, and upper back look and feel.) Full sit-ups can also be harmful if you have lower back pain because they put pressure on that area.

4. If an exercise or position reduces your pain, it is probably beneficial. If it causes pain, it is harmful and you should not do it. Trust the feedback you get from your body.

5. At one time most physicians in this country considered arching the lower back to be harmful and rounding it to be beneficial. Therefore, flexion exercises (knees-to-chest) were the type most frequently given to back patients. It is now recognized that the ability to round *and* arch the lower back is necessary for a healthy spine, and that both motions should be included in an exercise program.

6. Since a lack of flexibility in the back muscles is a frequent companion to back pain, exercises that stretch and limber are as important as those that strengthen. If your muscles are tense most of the time, you should include at least one exercise in which you practice mental and physical relaxation.

7. Last, but important, your exercise program should be enjoyable and not be so long and time consuming that somehow you never get around to doing it. Exercising should fit comfortably into your life-style and work schedule.

SHOULD YOU EXERCISE WHEN YOUR BACK HURTS?

No. If you are in pain, you should not do your regular exercise program. A hurting back is telling you that it needs special attention.

Lie down and rest as much as possible, in whatever position gives you the most relief. Try lying on your back with pillows under your knees. This position reduces pain for most people.

While you are resting your back, practice the breathing exercise in Chapter 8. I also suggest that you go through the movement sequence in Chapter 9 as an effective way of keeping back spasm from getting worse.

The cardinal rule when your back hurts is to be extremely conscientious about maintaining good spinal alignment as you sit and move around. After your back gets better you can return to your regular exercise program.

USING GYM EQUIPMENT

Exercising with weights (or any form of equipment designed to give resistance) works *all* the skeletal muscles, not just the ones you are specifically strengthening. The other muscles automatically start working to stabilize the body—that is, to keep the rest of your body in place while you work on one area. Stabilization is a normal muscle function and helps the body work efficiently.

If your overall use of your body is not correct, however, the extra stabilizing can hurt your back by exaggerating poor postural habits. For example, if you habitually compress your spine, the compression will be greatly increased as you lift weights or work against resistance.

Following are some ways to protect your back when you use resistive equipment:

Knee Straightening and Knee Bending Exercises (Sitting)

Have a firm support behind you to keep from slumping, or use your back muscles to keep your spine lengthened. The weight should not be so heavy that it forces you to take your spine out of good vertical alignment.

Arm and Shoulder Girdle Exercises

Think of your spine lengthening up between your shoulder blades (or of lengthening out through the top of your head if you are lying down).

Rowing Machine

Do not let the upper and lower back round completely as you lean forward and pull back. Keep enough tone in the back muscles so your back maintains length, and do most of your leaning forward from the hip joints.

Curl-Ups and Other Exercises That Round the Back

The way you return to the starting position is as important as the curl-up itself. You should finish each repetition by returning your spine to its fully lengthened state and your chest and shoulders to an open and "widened" position. Some zealous exercisers like to work the abdominal muscles in the mid-range of a curl-up in order to increase endurance. I am not partial to this practice, but if you are, think of lengthening your spine into the curve as you work.

Stationary Bicycle

You can either sit upright or lean your torso forward from your hip joints while supporting yourself with your arms (place your hands where the handlebars meet in front). Either position is fine as long as you maintain length in your torso. Your pelvis should move slightly as your legs move; however, do not let it drop down in a side-to-side motion or you will strain your lower back and sacroiliac joints. As you pedal, think of your knees releasing forward from your pelvis.

As I let my eyes sweep over a gym full of eager people energetically pulling and pushing on machines, I see that necks, shoulders, and upper backs are the body areas most consistently misaligned. Modern exercise equipment is, for the most part, designed to give good support to the lower back, but the needs of the upper back and neck are not considered. As you work, therefore, give yourself the instructions to let your head lead your spine into length and your shoulders release out to the sides.

A DAILY EXERCISE PROGRAM

I have found the following exercises form a good basic program for people with back, neck, and shoulder pain. There are limbering exercises, which are aimed at restoring normal mobility to the spine and back. The strengthening exercises, which reinforce the "corseting" function of the torso muscles, are the kind that encourage good postural support. The final exercise is for relaxation. If you wish to add other exercises, use the guidelines I have given you when you make your selection.

Try to exercise *at least once a day*. When you need to gain strength and mobility you must exercise daily because progress results from the cumulative effect of exercising regularly. If you can fit twice a day into your schedule, your progress will be faster. Later, when your aim is simply to maintain the strength and mobility you already have, you can exercise every other day if you prefer.

If any of the exercises make your back feel particularly good, do not hesitate to repeat them as often as your body feels the need. For example, many people feel better every time they do the knee circles or the back and shoulder stretches.

1: Training the Abdominal Muscles While Standing

Purpose: To train the abdominal muscles to support the lower back. You should do this important exercise frequently during the day. (Try to remember to do it any time you are standing in line.) Gradually these muscles will get accustomed to giving more support. This exercise will be incorporated into many of the ones that follow.

Starting position: Stand profile to a mirror (you will not need the mirror after you learn the exercise).

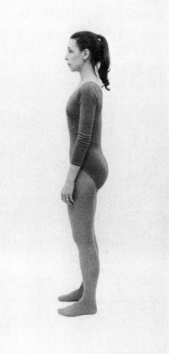

Instructions: Gently tighten the lower abdominal muscles (below the navel) sufficiently to decrease the arch in your lower back, and hold for 5 counts. Lengthen your entire spine while tightening and maintain that length when releasing. You can check to see if you are doing the exercise correctly by placing your hand just below your belly button so that you can feel the muscles contract.

Repeat 10 times.

This exercise should be done gently, not vigorously. Use the mirror to check the lengthening and alignment of your spine.

2: Balancing

Purpose: To train the abdominal and back muscles to support and lengthen the spine.

Starting position: Stand with feet 3 to 4 inches apart.

Instructions: Think of your head and spine lengthening up as you tighten your lower abdominal muscles. Maintain this tightening as you raise one knee up in front and hold for 5 counts.

Repeat, raising the other knee.

Alternate sides total of 10 times (5 each side).

Notice how your balance improves when you think of your head and spine lengthening up.

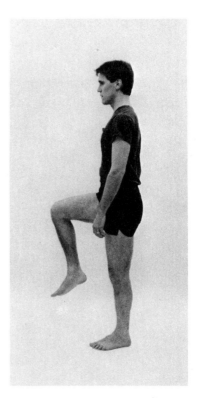

3: Training the Abdominal Muscles While Walking

Purpose: To train the abdominal muscles to work during activity.

Instructions: Walk around the room, gently tightening your lower abdominal muscles for 4 steps, then releasing for 4 steps. Think of your head and spine lengthening up the entire time. The tightening should not interfere with normal leg and arm motion.

Repeat the sequence 5 times.

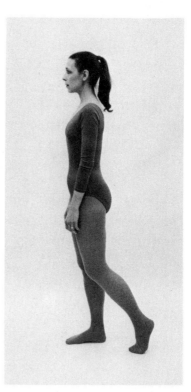

You should also do this exercise occasionally while walking outside.

4: Side Bending

Purpose: To limber the back and strengthen the side torso muscles. This exercise is excellent as preparation for returning to active sports.

Starting position: Take a comfortably wide stance (feet at least 12 inches apart).

Instructions: Slowly bend to the right side while raising your left arm out to the side and then overhead. Tighten abdominal muscles to support your lower back throughout the exercise and give your motion a flowing quality. Think of your spine lengthening as you move.

Repeat to the left side, raising your right arm.

Alternate sides for a total of 10 times (5 each side).

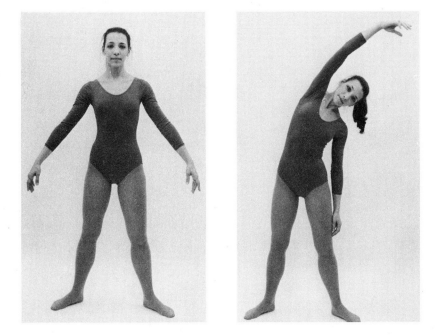

5: Rotation

Purpose: To limber the spine. Since spinal rotation is needed for most sports, this is a good preparatory exercise for returning to sports after an episode of back pain.

Starting position: Take a comfortably wide stance (feet at least 12 inches apart).

Instructions: Rotate your head and torso to the right to look behind you while letting your left heel come off the floor. Use your abdominal muscles to support your lower back and move in a flowing manner. You will feel your entire spine, from your neck down, gently rotating.

Repeat to the left side, letting your right heel come off the floor.

Alternate sides for a total of 10 times (5 each side).

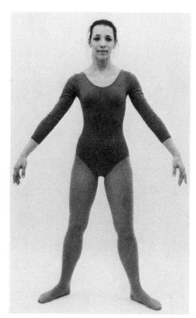 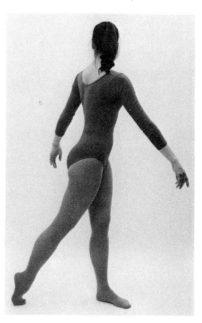

6: Balancing on Hands and Knees

Purpose: To strengthen the back muscles.

Starting position: On hands and knees. Place knees hip-width apart. Look at the floor throughout this exercise so the back of your neck can lengthen.

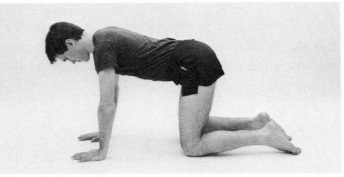

Instructions: Raise your right arm and left leg about 10 inches off floor and hold for 5 counts.

Repeat, raising your left arm and right leg.

Alternate sides for a total of 10 times (5 each side).

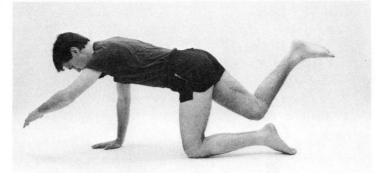

Notice how your balance improves as you think of lengthening out through the top of your head.

7: Crawling

Purpose: To gently limber the lower back.

Starting position: On hands and knees. Look down at the floor throughout this exercise so the back of your neck can lengthen.

Instructions: Slowly crawl forward a few steps and then crawl backward. (Use whatever sequence of hand-knee motion that comes naturally.) Be aware of the gentle motion that occurs throughout your spine and pelvis.

Repeat the forward and back sequence 3 times.

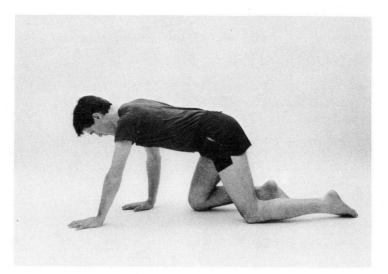

8: Cat Exercise

Purpose: To limber the lower back.

Starting position: On hands and knees. Place knees hip-width apart. Look down at the floor so the back of your neck can lengthen.

Instructions: Alternately round and arch your lower back, doing the motion gently and only as far as feels comfortable. To encourage your lower spine to move, think of the area below your navel moving.

Repeat 6 times (rounding and arching equals 1 count).

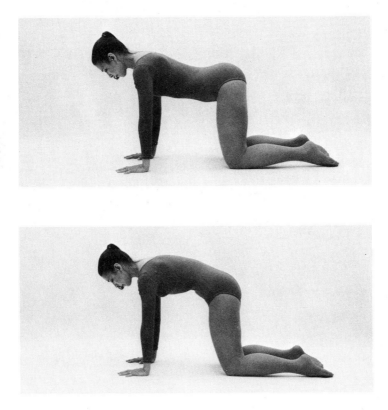

9: Donkey Tail Exercise

Purpose: To limber the spine.

Starting position: On hands and knees. Place knees hip-width apart.

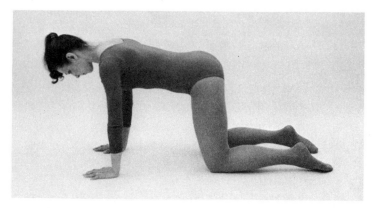

Instructions: Bend your torso gently to the right side and look behind you as if you were an animal looking at its tail. Bend only as far as is comfortable.

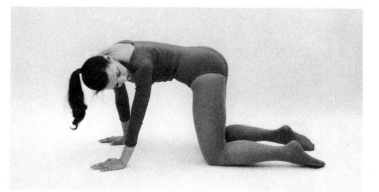

Repeat, bending to the left.

Alternate sides for a total of 8 times (4 each side).

10: Fold-Up Resting Position

Purpose: To stretch the lower back. This is an excellent position to rest in when your lower back feels tired or tight.

Starting Position: Assume the position shown in the picture. The tops of your feet should be against the floor, your buttocks should be close to or resting on your heels, and your entire torso should be draped forward with your forehead and arms resting on the floor.

Instructions: Stay in this position a few minutes while breathing in a relaxed way. If your knees and feet are uncomfortable, remain in the position only briefly. Gradually you will become more limber.

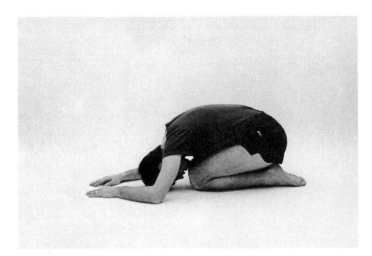

Important note for back-lying exercises: If your head tilts backwards when you are lying on your back, place a pillow or book under your head thick enough to eliminate the backward tilt.

11: Knee Circles

Purpose: To limber a tight lower back.

Starting position: Lie on your back with both knees up toward your chest; place a hand on each knee.

Instructions: Slowly make 5 small circles with your knees, separating them and then bringing them together. You will feel your pelvis gently rocking.

Gently pull both knees as close to your chest as is comfortable and hold for 5 counts.

Repeat the sequence 5 times.

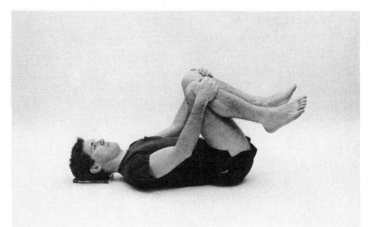

Most people do this exercise with too much tension in their shoulders and arms. To avoid this, think of your shoulders releasing out to the sides throughout the exercise.

12: Pelvic Tilt with Leg Extended

Purpose: To strengthen abdominal and front thigh muscles.

Starting position: Lie on your back with both knees bent and feet on floor.

Instructions: Tighten the abdominal muscles (but not your buttocks) so that your back flattens against the floor. (You will feel your head and spine lengthening out.) Hold your abdominal muscles tight throughout the next 3 steps.

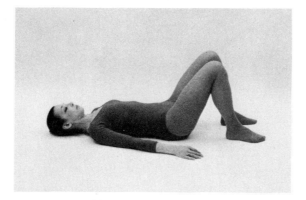

Bring the right knee to your chest. (You will feel your head and spine lengthening even more.)

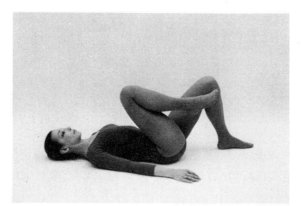

Straighten the right leg out, keeping it slightly off the floor. (You will feel your abdominal muscles working harder to keep your back flat on the floor.)

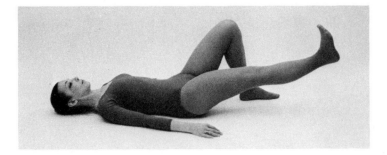

Bring the right knee to your chest again.

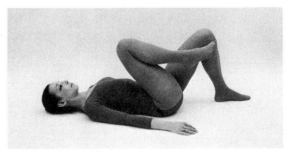

Return the right leg to the starting position and relax the abdominal muscles.

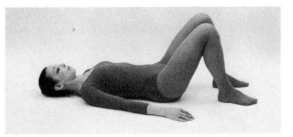

Repeat the entire sequence with left leg.

Alternate sides for a total of 10 times (5 each side).

13: Modified Bicycle

Purpose: To stretch the hamstrings and hip muscles.

Starting position: Lie on your back with both knees up toward your chest. Hold the left knee with both hands.

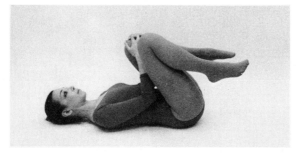

Instructions: Straighten your right leg up in the air with your foot at right angles to your leg. (You will feel a stretch in back of the leg.)

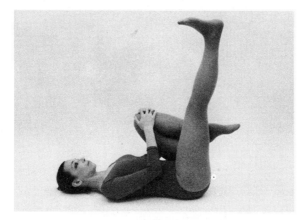

Keeping the knee straight, lower the right leg to the floor and hold position for 5 counts.

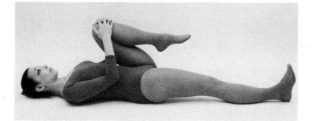

Raise the right leg up again, still keeping the knee straight. (You will feel your abdominal and front thigh muscles working hard.)

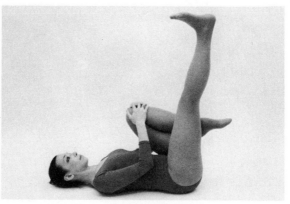

Return the right leg to the starting position.

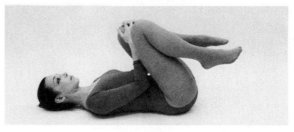

Repeat entire sequence with left leg.

Alternate sides for a total of 10 times (5 each side).

14: Abdominal Exercise

Purpose: To strengthen the abdominal muscles.

Starting position: Sit with your knees bent and feet on the floor. Fold your arms in front of your chest.

Instructions: Lean your entire torso slightly back until you feel your abdominal muscles working. Hold this position for 5 counts while thinking of your head and spine lengthening up. Return to starting position by coming forward.

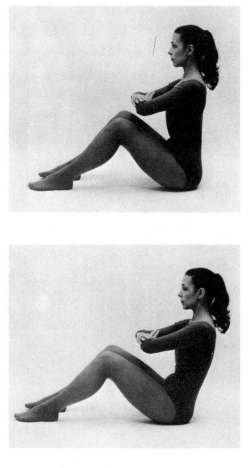

You will not feel strain in your neck as you lean back if you continue to look straight ahead instead of up at the ceiling. Occasionally turn your head while leaning back to be sure you are not tightening your neck.

Repeat 5 times.

15: Prone Arm and Leg Raise

Purpose: To strengthen back and shoulder blade muscles.

Starting position: Lie face down with two pillows under your stomach and arms overhead, resting on floor. Your forehead is on the floor.

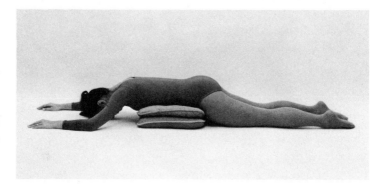

Instructions: Raise your right arm and left leg *slightly* off the floor (4 to 5 inches), and hold for 5 counts. Let your head rest on the floor throughout.

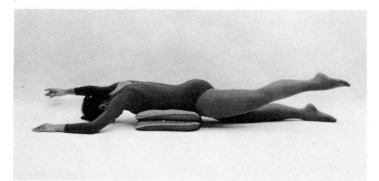

Alternate sides total of 10 times (5 times each side).

16: Hip Raise

Purpose: To strengthen back and buttock muscles.

Starting position: Lie on your back with knees bent up and feet on floor.

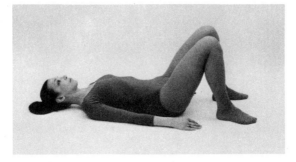

Instructions: Raise your hips slightly off the floor and hold for 4 counts. Then slowly lower them.

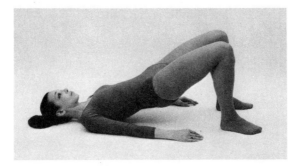

Repeat 10 times.

17: Knees Side to Side

Purpose: To limber hip joints and lower back. (This exercise has two versions. The first provides a stretch, and the second strengthens the abdominal muscles as well. You can benefit from doing both.)

VERSION 1

Starting position: Lie on your back with knees bent up and feet on floor.

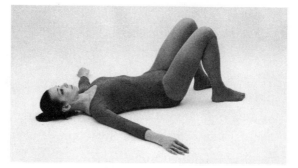

Instructions: Slowly lower both knees toward the floor on the right side as far as they can go comfortably. Relax in this position for a minute. You may find that your knees drop closer to the floor as you relax into the stretch. Raise your knees to the starting position and slowly lower them to the other side.

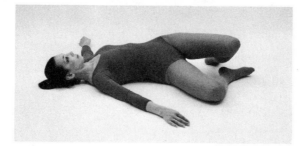

Alternate sides 10 times (5 times each side).

VERSION 2

Starting position: Lie on your back with knees up toward your chest and arms out to the sides at shoulder level, resting on floor.

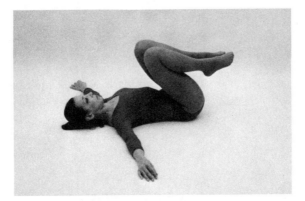

Instructions: Slowly lower both knees to the floor on the right side and rest in this position a moment. Use the abdominal muscles to help raise your knees up to the starting position and lower them to the other side.

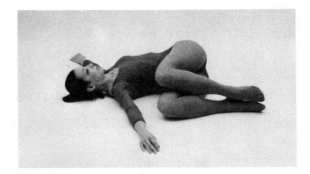

Alternate sides 10 times (5 each side).

18: Leg Raise

Purpose: To stretch hamstrings and strengthen front thigh muscles.

Starting position: Lie on your back. Bend the left knee up, keeping your foot on the floor. The right leg is straight.

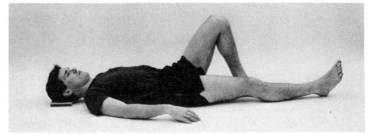

Instructions: Gently tighten your abdominal muscles so that your back is flat against the floor. Then raise your right leg up in the air as far as possible while keeping the knee straight and the foot at a right angle to the leg. Think of the hamstring muscles (in back of thigh) releasing into the stretch.

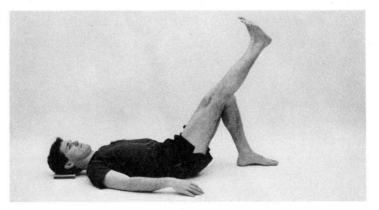

Raise and lower one leg 10 times; then repeat with other leg. Your abdominals should work throughout the sequence.

Repeat this sequence 3 times.

19: Arm Circle Rotation

Purpose: To limber the spine and shoulders. Daily practice will increase your flexibility, making the exercise easier.

Starting position: Lie on your left side with your knees bent comfortably up toward your chest and your arms straight out in front on the floor. Some people are more comfortable with a pillow under the head.

Instructions: Keeping your hand on the floor as much as possible, slowly circle your right arm up toward your head and around your body, letting your head and shoulders follow your arm. Continue until your arm has made a complete circle and is back at the starting point. (You can pretend that you are drawing a large circle around your body with a piece of chalk.)

It is all right for your knees to come up off the floor slightly. When you are in the diagonal or rotated position you will feel a stretch in the front of your shoulder, across your chest, and in your lower back.

Repeat 8 times.

Roll over and repeat.

This is one of my favorite exercises because it feels wonderful and gives a good stretch to the shoulders and front chest area. It is also a good rotation exercise to do for two weeks following a period of inactivity due to back pain, before returning to sports.

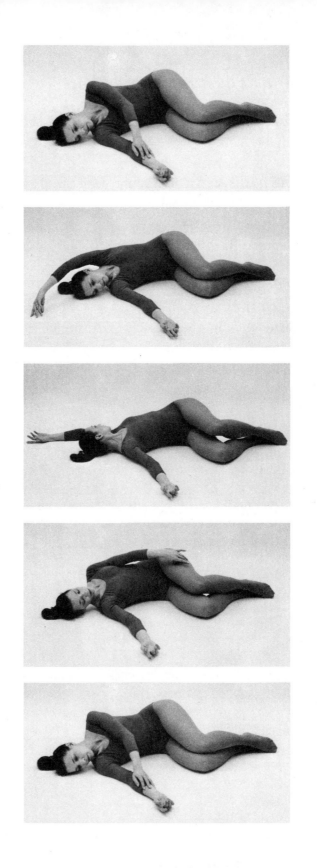

20: Upper Back Stretch (Sitting in Chair)

Purpose: To improve spinal alignment and shoulder placement.

Starting position: Sit in a chair near the front edge, with your back lengthened and arms at your sides.

Instructions: Raise both arms out to the sides and up overhead. Then bend your elbows so your forearms drape gently on top of your head.

With forearms on your head, gently stretch your head and spine up toward the ceiling. (Keep looking straight ahead, do *not* tilt your head back.) You will feel a stretch in your upper back.

Straighten your arms up toward the ceiling, and then lower them out to the sides and all the way down. As you lower your arms, think of your head and spine lengthening up. (This part of the exercise reminds me of a corkscrew with the arms that go down as the cork goes up.)

Repeat 4 times.

This is a good exercise to do every half hour if you work at a desk for long periods of time. It will prevent fatigue building up in your shoulders and back and remind you not to slump over your work.

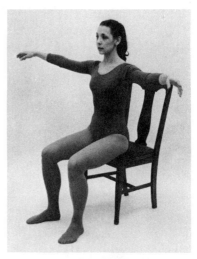

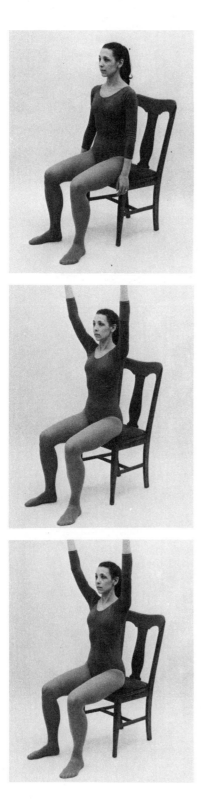

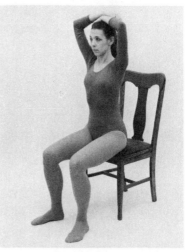

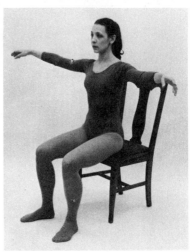

21: *Relaxation*

Lie on your back (in bed or on the floor) with pillows under your knees and a small pillow under your head. Close your
eyes and think of relaxing all your muscles, beginning with
your forehead and face and working your way down to your
toes.

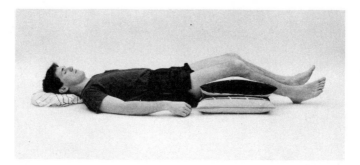

While relaxing throughout your body, mentally review the
four Concepts of Good Use:

*Let your neck release so your head can balance forward and
out.* (Use the words "forward and *out*" when you are lying
down.)

Let your torso release into length and width.

Let your legs release away from your pelvis.

Let your shoulders release out to the sides.

I also recommend that you do the breathing exercise described in Chapter 8.

Spending twenty to thirty minutes a day relaxing your mind
and body will help your back heal and increase your ability
to get rid of tension.

12

Concerning Running, Swimming, Golf and Other Sports

"This is exactly how I am supposed to align my spine when playing golf."

"My tennis instructor has been trying to get me to use my back and shoulders this way for a year."

"This is exactly the way I am supposed to bend my knees and align my spine when skiing."

THOSE OF MY PATIENTS who enjoy golf, tennis, and skiing frequently remark on the similarity between what is considered correct form for these sports and the Concepts of Good Use. The ones who have applied the Alexander Technique to sports have improved their skills greatly.

The basic principles for using your body correctly are the same whether you are playing tennis, playing the violin, or picking up the baby. Your body will have increased strength, coordination, and efficiency when you use it in a way that allows your muscles to release and your head to lead your spine into length.

You can help train your muscles to work efficiently during any activity by thinking of the Concepts of Good Use:

Allow your neck to release so your head can balance forward and up.
Allow your torso to release into length and width.
Allow your legs to release away from your pelvis.
Allow your shoulders to release out to the sides.

If you have a competitive nature and are playing a competitive sport, the Concepts will help you in another way. They will enable you to stay in touch with your body so you can prevent the tensions of the game from going into your back.

RETURNING TO SPORTS

Participating in a sport on a regular basis will be tremendously beneficial for your back and your morale. When a back problem has kept you from your favorite sport, and your physician or physical therapist has finally given you the go-ahead to return, you will need to take steps to protect your back. Here are some suggestions:

1. Play for short periods at first. Gradually increase your playing time as you build up endurance.

2. Do a warm-up and gentle stretch before playing and a more vigorous stretch and cool down afterwards. You will be able to stretch more thoroughly when your body is well warmed up. Use a sustained pull; do not bounce.

3. Include the Standing Rotation Exercise (exercise 5 in Chapter 11) in your daily exercise program for at least two weeks before returning to sports, and then make it a regular part of your warm-up. Since almost all sports require spinal rotation (picture the batter in baseball, the golfer, the tennis player), you will need to prepare for play by improving spinal flexibility.

4. Remember that the back you take with you onto the tennis court or golf course is the same one you have at your desk or in the car. Therefore, your back will be in better shape for sports if you protect it by keeping it lengthened at other times.

HOW SPECIFIC SPORTS AFFECT YOUR BACK

You may be unsure which sports can help or harm your back. Following are some pros and cons of various athletic activities, to help you decide which to start, which to continue, and which to stop.

Aerobic Exercise Classes

In my opinion, aerobic exercise classes can be harmful to the back and legs because of all the jumping. If you do attend a class that involves a lot of jumping, apply a strong "up" thought to your head and torso so that your spine gets good support from your torso muscles. Be sure you do not throw your head back or your neck will be compressed with every jump. An alternative is to seek out one of the newly popular "low impact" aerobics classes, which require little or no jumping.

Biking

Riding a bicycle is an excellent way to exercise the entire body. No matter what style of bike you use, it is most important to maintain length in your spine. (Some doctors recommend sitting upright if you have back trouble.) Let your shoulders release out to the sides—think of releasing out along your collar bones—and let your legs release forward, away from your hips, as you pedal.

If you use a bike with curl-under handlebars, be sure to lengthen the back of your neck occasionally by looking down or to the side.

Golf

To align your spine correctly at address, incline your torso forward from the hip joints, not from the waist, and do not round

your upper back. You will find it helpful to practice your alignment while standing in profile to a mirror.

Since golf requires a strong rotatory motion in the torso, it is
important to keep your spine lengthened and your hip joints
released. A smoother rotation can then take place from your hip
joints up through your torso, instead of being concentrated in one
area of your back.

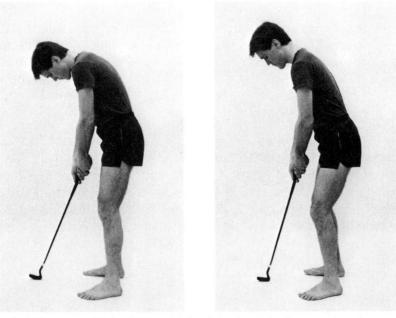

(Left) **Incorrect.** *(Right)* **Correct: Maintaining length in the torso gives the arms
more power and protects the back when the body rotates during a full golf swing.**

Running

When asked to recommend athletic activities that are good for
the body and back, I do not include running because it is hard on
the back, legs, and feet. Did you know that every running step
loads your weight-bearing joints with two and a half times your
body weight? A few of my patients have found race walking a good
alternative because it is as accessible as running and provides the
same aerobic and weight-control benefits while being kinder to
the body.

If you feel that running is the one activity you can get yourself
to do on a regular basis, and that to discontinue would severely
compromise your sense of well-being, do it with care. Be sure to

give yourself the instructions to lengthen your entire spine and let your legs move freely forward from the hip joints. Your torso muscles will be able to give your spine good support and your legs and feet will be more correctly aligned.

Do not forget to stretch your calf muscles and front and back thigh muscles before and after running.

Skiing

I would not advise you to take up downhill skiing as a beginner if you have a history of serious back trouble. Cross country skiing is a better choice because it is less hazardous for the back. If, however, you are already an accomplished skier and your back has been declared stable by your physician, I see no reason why you should not ski again.

Downhill skiing involves rotation throughout the body, with the torso rotating against the legs. You need to maintain as much rotation as possible in the hip joints so you do not strain the lower back. Think of your legs releasing away from your pelvis as you swivel.

Skiing with correct form is an excellent way of practicing good use of your back since it trains you to keep your spine lengthened while your knees are bent.

Swimming

This is an excellent activity for people with back problems. The water minimizes the pressure of gravity while offering enough resistance to exercise the entire body. A key to ease while swimming is to think of allowing the water to totally support your torso while you use your arms and legs to propel yourself forward. I recommend that you try different swimming strokes to see how they feel. The back and side strokes are easiest on the back.

There are many ways to exercise in water. Holding onto a kickboard while you work your legs provides good exercise for both the torso and leg muscles. You can minimize arching of the lower back when you are on your stomach by placing the kickboard far enough under your body. You can also stand in the water, holding on to the side of the pool, and do exercises to strengthen your legs and abdominal muscles.

Tennis

Many of my patients play tennis, and they have been able to return to this wonderful sport without a recurrence of back problems. I have also known those with a history of back pain to take up tennis as a new sport. They have not had problems either.

It is important to give top priority to maintaining correct use of your back as you play. Be particularly careful to keep as much length in your spine as possible when you serve.

Released hip joints are also extremely important. Not only will your back be protected by being in good alignment, but your agility on the court will increase. Released hip joints will enable you to change directions more easily, run faster, and respond more quickly to your choice of forehand or backhand.

You will discover that the instructions for correct use of your back are in harmony with those for correct playing form. Shrugging your shoulders or pulling them forward when you hit the ball are examples of faulty habits that prevent your arms from getting power from the large muscles in your back.

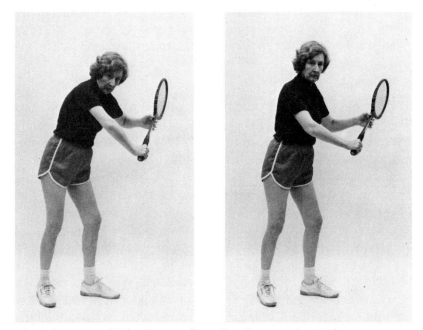

(Left) Incorrect. *(Right)* Correct: **Rounding the upper back takes power away from the arms and increases the likelihood of injuring the back.**

Walking

If the more active sports are not to your liking or are not medically appropriate, a regular walking program will benefit your back by keeping your entire body "tuned up." Walk for twenty minutes at least three times a week. Maintain a brisk pace that is both comfortable and invigorating. Be particularly observant of your spinal alignment when increasing your pace for cardiovascular benefit. Do not pull your head back and down or push your chest forward.

My main concern is not so much which sports you choose, as how well you use your body while you engage in each sport. You should select activities you enjoy, and then keep your mind focused on what you are doing instead of letting your thoughts wander off. Making use of the four Concepts of Good Use will keep your thoughts correctly focused, protect your back, and increase both your playing pleasure and skill.

13
SCOLIOSIS

THE HUMAN RACE is well-served, for the most part, by research that transforms yesterday's medical mysteries into today's curable ailments. One of the conditions that continues to defy this happy progression is scoliosis.

Scoliosis (the Greek word for crookedness) is a condition in which the spine has a lateral (sideways) curvature. Doctors have identified the causes of some types of scoliosis, such as an incompletely formed vertebra, or muscle spasticity in those who have cerebral palsy. But the most common form is called *idiopathic* scoliosis, which means that the cause is unknown.

There are a few facts that are known about idiopathic scoliosis. The condition frequently runs in families. Four out of five children with scoliosis severe enough to require treatment will be girls. If scoliosis is going to become worse, it usually happens most rapidly during adolescence, the fast-growing years. The vertebrae in the area of the spine where the curve occurs become wedge-shaped and rotate.

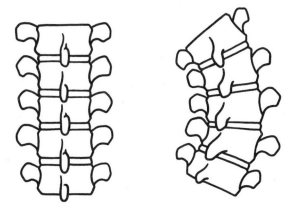

(Left) **Normally shaped vertebrae.** *(Right)* **Wedge-shaped vertebrae characteristic of scoliosis.**

Unfortunately, there is no way to predict how far each individual spine will curve to the side during the growing years. In some adolescents the curvature progresses very slowly, stabilizes when still slight, and never requires treatment other than the same considerate attention everyone's back deserves—good postural habits and enough exercise to keep the torso muscles strong. In others, the curve progresses steadily until the possibility of deformity and health impairment necessitates the use of a brace. If the brace does not stop the progression, surgical stabilization of the spine is usually recommended.

Once skeletal growth is complete, the curvature usually stabilizes. In some cases, though, a curve has continued to progress slowly over a number of years after the growth period. And in a very few cases, a sudden and severe increase in the curvature has occurred in an adult, making surgical stabilization advisable. Although scoliosis is usually not painful during adolescence, it can sometimes precipitate arthritic or muscle pain in adults who have a relatively severe curve.

The importance of early detection, so that each child can be watched and appropriate treatment given, has now been recognized.

In many schools throughout the country, children are routinely examined for scoliosis by a nurse or other trained personnel.

Parents frequently question whether poor postural habits cause scoliosis in the growing child. The answer is no, there is no direct causal relationship between posture and idiopathic scoliosis. Well-meaning parents do not need to impose guilt and fear on their children by telling them that if they do not sit and stand properly, they will develop scoliosis. Nevertheless, anyone who has idiopathic scoliosis will find that good postural habits and a more efficient use of the body can improve appearance, increase physical comfort, and encourage a more positive self-concept by improving body image.

BENEFITS OF THE ALEXANDER TECHNIQUE

If you have scoliosis, the Alexander Technique can teach you how to use your back in a way that keeps it strong and as well-balanced as possible. The technique should be used as an addition to, not a replacement for, medical supervision and treatment. Particularly with the growing child, periodic medical checkups by a physician who is knowledgeable about scoliosis are essential.

Many adults have said to me, "Even though my X-rays remain the same, I can see that my posture is getting worse, that my curve is becoming more noticeable than it was a few years ago." To this I respond, "Let us work for a while with the Alexander Technique. It will help you identify and eliminate postural habits that are making your back look less symmetrical." Because the shoulder girdle, rib cage, and muscles and ligaments of the torso are flexible, a person's postural appearance can, indeed, change— for better or worse—while the degree of lateral curvature of the spine remains the same.

Many adolescents with scoliosis have told me that they dislike their bodies and feel betrayed by them. I work with these teenagers in front of a mirror so they can see how much better they look as they lengthen their spines and release their shoulders out to the sides. The Alexander Technique is an extremely effective way of improving self-image.

Those who have had a spinal fusion often believe they have no postural choices. However, unless the entire spine has been fused, some flexibility remains and using it to achieve more spinal lengthening can mean the difference between having or not having back pain. Even when the entire spine has been fused, the Concepts of Good Use can be helpful for increasing ease of movement and reducing pain caused by unnecessary muscle tension.

PATIENTS' STORIES

Following are a few of the experiences I have had using the Alexander Technique with my scoliosis patients. After I tell you their stories, I will instruct you, as I do them, in the ways you can work by yourself to improve the comfort and appearance of your back.

Anne

About ten years ago an orthopedist referred Anne, then age forty-one, to me for Alexander lessons. Anne had a severe "S-shaped" scoliosis with each curve over 60 degrees, and she was suffering from intermittent numbness in one arm and hand, lower and upper back pain, and pain referred from her lower back into both legs. She also tired easily and suffered from shortness of breath. She had worn a brace for two years as a teenager, but had not had any other treatment.

Over a twelve-month period, during which Anne took lessons once a week, her pain disappeared and her torso began to look more symmetrical. Her X-rays remained essentially the same except for a 4-degree improvement in the upper curve and an increase in the spaces between the ribs on the more compressed left side. These changes are consistent with an improvement in Anne's breathing that enabled her to get through the day without feeling exhausted and climb stairs without becoming breathless.

Anne had an interesting experience related to her appearance. To mask the asymmetry in her shoulders and back, she had most of her clothing made to order. Shortly before starting Alexander lessons, she had ordered several fall outfits from her regular dressmaker. When she picked up the finished clothing three months later, nothing fit as expected. The dressmaker was extremely upset, believing she had made a mistake in measuring and cutting the clothing.

Anne finally realized what had happened. In response to the lessons, her body had changed so much that the dressmaker's measurements were no longer accurate! Since it seemed likely that her body would continue to change, Anne decided to postpone ordering new clothes. A year later the dressmaker made new measurements. When Anne and I compared the two sets (see chart), we found an increase of two inches from shoulder to waist, both in front and in back, and an increase of one inch in shoulder width. Anne's shoulders were now level, and her waist had decreased by two inches with no change in her weight.

ANNE'S MEASUREMENTS

BODY PART	BEFORE ALEXANDER	AFTER ALEXANDER
Shoulder to waist	13 1/2" back 14 1/2" front	15 1/2" back 16 1/2" back
Shoulders (width)	15 1/2"	16 1/2"
Bust	37 1/2"	38"
Waist	33"	31"
Hips	40"	39 1/2"
Waist to floor	41 1/2"	43"
Crotch to floor	31"	32 3/4"
Arm length, right	37 1/2"	37 1/2"
Arm length, left	37"	37 1/2"

Ruth

Ruth was forty-eight years old when her orthopedist referred her to me for Alexander lessons. She had a moderate "S-shaped" scoliosis, with each curve approximately 40 degrees.

I went to Ruth's home for the first two sessions because her back was in such acute spasm that she could not get out of bed. She told me that her episodes of disabling back spasm were occurring with increasing frequency.

Over the following ten years, I worked with Ruth intermittently. The results have been dramatic. Even though she was at an age when women have normal spinal changes that, combined with scoliosis, often result in increasing back pain, Ruth's back pain is gone! Moreover, her appearance is greatly improved. She started taking tennis lessons for the first time when she was fifty-five, and golf when she was fifty-seven. Ruth has been able to enjoy these sports with no recurrence of back pain.

Judy

When Judy, age fourteen, came with her parents for her first visit, she knew I had something to do with posture and therefore put on her best posture performance for the "before" photograph I take of all my teenage patients. Later in the visit, as I was talking to her mother, Judy's mind wandered and she adopted a very different stance. When I remarked on it she told me that this was her favorite way of standing and agreed to stay in that position while I photographed her again.

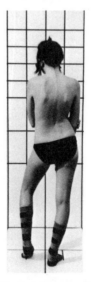

Judy's favorite standing posture emphasizes her curvature.

Judy's scoliosis consisted of a single curve to the left in the lower spine, which was exaggerated by her "favorite" standing posture. Her practice was to bend her left knee so that the left side of her pelvis dipped down lower than the right, causing her spine to curve even farther to the left. I found that Judy's habitual sitting posture also increased the extent to which her lower spine curved to the left.

I explained to Judy that she could improve both the look and strength of her back by eliminating those postural habits that "feed into" her scoliosis. Compare the picture taken during her first visit with the picture taken four months later. In the later photograph Judy's head is more centered (instead of tilted to the right), her back has more length, and her shoulders are more level. Other important changes are that her upper back is less rounded and her entire torso is better balanced. Also compare how her arms hang: in the earlier picture her right arm is closer to the body than her left, while later they are hanging more symmetrically.

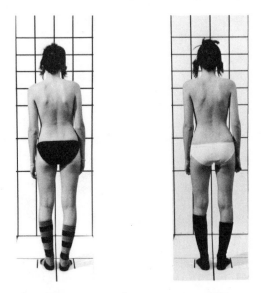

(Left) Judy before starting Alexander lessons. *(Right)* Judy after four months of lessons. Notice that her shoulders are more level, her head is more centered, and her back has more length.

Sheila

The two photographs of Sheila also illustrate the improvement typical of those who apply the Alexander Technique to their postural habits. The photo on the left was taken at the time of Sheila's initial visit. The one on the right was taken six months later.

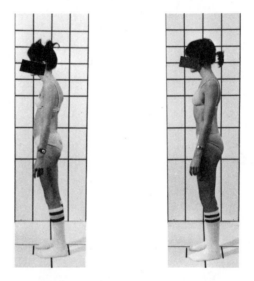

Both Judy and Sheila have moderate curves and are being checked every three months by an orthopedist. The "being watched" stage (to see whether a curve is going to stabilize or progess to the point where a brace is required) is an excellent time for an adolescent to study the Alexander Technique, to learn that there are postural choices and to see in the mirror the difference these choices make.

WORKING ON YOUR OWN

Of particular importance, if you have scoliosis, is that your postural habits support your spine in as much length as possible. They should not feed into your curvature. Compare the two photographs at the top of the next page. In the right-hand picture, the shoulders are more level, and the arms are hanging more symmetrically (an indication that the torso is better balanced).

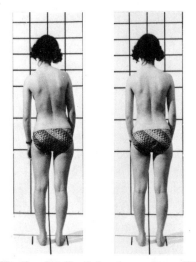

(Left) **Posturally "feeding into" a lateral curvature.** *(Right)* **Head and spine lengthening up. Notice that the back is better aligned and the shoulders are more level.**

Use a mirror to help increase your awareness of what you want to change. Postural habits become so automatic that most of us are unaware of them until our mirror alerts us to their existence. You will also find it helpful to have a clear mental picture of the location and direction of the lateral curve or curves in your spine.

Those of you with scoliosis in the part of your spine where your ribs attach should know which way your rib cage tends to rotate. For example, if your upper (thoracic) spine curves to the right, the right side of your rib cage will tend to rotate toward the back and the left side toward the front. Please don't hesitate to ask your doctor or physical therapist to give you this information, because it will help you recognize and avoid habits of use that emphasize your scoliosis.

As you follow the instructions for working on your own, you will see that they incorporate Alexander's four basic Concepts of Good Use. You should supplement the instructions with those in Chapter 7, "Positions We All Get Into."

Sitting Correctly

Place a chair facing the mirror and sit in your usual, most relaxed, way. Notice whether you are allowing your torso to slump
sideways into your curvature.

Here is how you can correct this tendency:

1. Think of your neck releasing so that your head can ease up
off your neck.

2. Think of your entire torso following the upward direction of
your head.

3. Change the way you are sitting so that your back has more
length. You may find it helpful to think of lengthening up equally
on both sides of your torso. If you want to lean against the back
of the chair for support, be sure you are sitting all the way back in
the seat with your pelvis squarely placed—not rotated to one side.

If you have one long lateral curvature in your spine, or one
curve that is considerably larger than the other, and your usual
way of sitting is to slump into that curve, you will feel the muscles next to the curve working harder than usual as you lengthen
your back. This is to be expected and does not mean you are doing anything wrong; your muscles are, indeed, working harder. As
your muscles gain strength and endurance from your efforts to sit
correctly, with your back lengthened, it will become easier. For
now, you can avoid overworking your muscles by thinking of
your back releasing into length and width, rather than thinking of
sitting up straight.

Keeping Your Shoulders Level

Again, sit in a chair facing the mirror in your usual, most relaxed way. Look at your shoulders in the mirror. If you have a
curve in the upper part of your spine that makes one shoulder
higher than the other, be sure you do not inadvertently increase
this difference when you are sitting. For example, if your right
shoulder is higher than the left, try not to lean your upper torso
to the left because that will make your right shoulder even higher.

You may be tempted to correct a higher right shoulder by leaning your torso to the right. This is not a good solution because it does not train your spine to be as lengthened as possible. Instead, adjust your sitting so that your spine has more length while you think of your head and spine lengthening up and your shoulders releasing out to the sides.

Here is an excellent exercise you can do any time during the day, either standing or sitting, to help your shoulders become more level (see exercise 20 in Chapter 11). When you watch yourself in the mirror as you do this exercise, you will see your shoulders become more symmetrical.

1. Extend both arms out to the sides and raise them overhead. Then bend your elbows so your forearms drape gently on top of your head.

2. Gently stretch your head and spine up into length, making sure not to tilt your head back.

3. Continue to lengthen your head and spine up as you slowly bring your arms out to the sides again, and down.

Keeping Your Head Centered

Use the mirror to check your head-neck alignment. The more you correct yourself, the sooner your head will feel "right" when it is centered, even though it will feel "wrong" at first.

I have noticed that both adults and teenagers have a tendency to hold their heads tilted to one side out of habit, even after a surgical fusion has reduced the severity of their curvatures. If you have had a spinal fusion, check in the mirror to see if this applies to you.

Carrying Your Purse or Briefcase

Stand in front of the mirror and hold your purse or briefcase the way you would if you were walking down the street. Are you raising one shoulder higher than the other and leaning slightly to one side?

Think of your spine lengthening up and your shoulders releasing out to the sides. Your spine will stay more centered and lengthened. It will be easier to align your head, neck, and back correctly if you use a purse with a long strap that goes across your torso.

Breathing More Efficiently

If you have a significant curve in your upper back, your ribs are more compressed on one side than on the other. Spend a few minutes every day doing the following exercise. It will help your rib cage become more flexible and symmetrical, which will make your breathing more efficient.

1. Face the mirror and place your hands on the sides of your rib cage just above the waist (thumbs toward the back, fingers toward the front).

2. Think of breathing equally into both hands. Breathe slowly and easily; do not take in more air than is comfortable. Watch your hands move with the in-and-out motion of your lower rib cage.

3. Think of your head and spine *continually* lengthening up as you breathe, and keep a mental image of your lower ribs moving freely out to the sides and in again.

Avoiding Rotation of the Rib Cage

Place a chair facing the mirror. Watch yourself move from sitting to standing, and back again. Notice whether your torso is "feeding into" your pattern of rotation *as you move*. Also notice if you are settling into the rotation when you get into your favorite sitting position.

You cannot correct the tendency to rotate into your curve by rotating in the opposite direction—you may overcorrect and compress your spine even more. You can avoid rotating your rib cage by thinking of your head leading your spine into length and your torso lengthening and widening.

If You Have Had a Spinal Fusion

Even if you have had a spinal fusion, you still have choices regarding your sitting and standing posture, particularly if any areas of your spine have not been fused. Experiment with how much you can lengthen your back or go into a slump while sitting, and again while standing. It will be much better for all the structures of your spine if you keep your torso muscles strong by maintaining a lengthened spine throughout the day.

PARTICULARLY FOR TEENAGERS

Ask your parents to put a long mirror in your room so that you can check your use of your head, neck, and torso whenever you like.

Talking on the Phone

Lie down when talking on the phone for a long time because it is easier on the back. You can lie on the floor or on your bed. Make yourself comfortable and be sure your spine is as lengthened as possible.

The other option is to sit up with your back lengthened and well-supported by a good chair, pillows, or the wall.

Carrying School Books

Stand in front of the mirror and hold your books the way you usually carry them. Check the alignment of your head and shoulders. Are you leaning to one side so that one shoulder is higher than the other? Experiment with other ways of carrying your books so that your head stays centered and your shoulders level. Using a knapsack on your back is a good idea. If you hang it on one shoulder, keep your spine lengthening and try to minimize the amount you lean to the side.

Practicing a Musical Instrument

Be aware of how you are using your back when you practice your musical instrument. When you think of your spine lengthen-

ing and your shoulders releasing out to the sides, you will be able
to play with less tension and more skill.

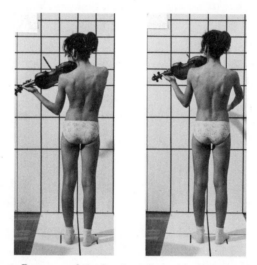

(Left) **Incorrect: Poor use of the head, neck, and back can accentuate a lateral
curvature and interfere with playing ability.** *(Right)* **Correct: Head leading up,
and back lengthening and widening, results in good spinal support and enhances
playing skill.**

Studying

Be aware of what positions you get into when you study. It's
better to study lying down than to sit slumped over, which is very
bad for your back.

If you like to sit on your bed to study, put a pillow behind you
to help keep your back lengthened. When you study at your desk
or at a table, you should have a good secretarial-type chair that
will encourage you to sit correctly. You may also be able to sit
with a more lengthened spine if you raise your working surface
slightly. It is better to raise your work up to you than to slump
down to it.

Many teenagers (and adults also) become so used to slumping
over their work that they feel they cannot write any other way.
Try to break yourself of this habit. You will discover that you can
write just as well with a lengthened back. If you have to get
closer to your work to see properly, do have your eyes checked.
Glasses may make it easier for you to sit correctly.

If You Wear a Brace

I am sure you have already heard this advice from your physical therapist: you should not collapse into your brace or lean against it.

Actively lengthen your spine frequently during the day so that your back and stomach muscles do not forget that their job is to hold you up. The exercises you have been given to keep your torso muscles strong while you must wear a brace are extremely important, but they will not *train* your muscles to support your spine properly when the brace is removed. The women I have worked with who wore a brace as teenagers have the same tendency to posturally "feed into" their curvatures as those who have never worn a brace. This tells me that the brace does not train you as far as your postural habits are concerned. Therefore, it is important for you to get used to supporting your own back *before* the brace is removed.

Spend a few minutes each day, when the brace is off, observing in the mirror how you can posturally support your spine to give it more length. While making your corrections, observe yourself from the front and also from the side.

Be Physically Active

I would like to encourage you to participate in any sports that appeal to you unless there is a medical reason not to. Dance classes would also be very beneficial. The more physically active you are, the better shape your back—as well as the rest of you—will be in.

14

The Performing Artist's Dilemma

PERFORMING ARTISTS were one of the first professional groups to recognize the value of Alexander's work. This is not surprising since Alexander, himself an actor, developed his technique as a solution to a dilemma experienced by many performers. Alexander found that the more he practiced his art form, the more his artistic potential was sabotaged by the practicing itself.

What makes the performer such a ready victim of this "practicing dilemma"? Practicing requires repetition. Although the purpose of this repetition is to develop skills that will enhance your innate talent, it works against you if you are also repeating—and therefore reinforcing—harmful habits of use.

Sometimes the consequences can be serious. A concert pianist came to see me with such severe shoulder pain she had not been able to practice for four months and, consequently, had to cancel concert engagements. A cellist was referred by her orthopedist with pain in her left shoulder that was interfering with her career. Violinists frequently suffer from neck and shoulder pain. Actors can develop serious voice trouble, as Alexander himself did. It is not uncommon for dancers to seriously injure their backs and knees.

Sometimes teachers inadvertently encourage poor use. One violinist I worked with had neck and shoulder pain as a direct result of poor early instruction. When he came for his first lesson, I noticed that his right shoulder was much lower than the left, and I asked him if he was aware of how compressed and tense it was. He said yes, and gave me the reason. When he was a child, his first violin teacher had not been able to break him of the habit of raising his shoulder when playing. The teacher finally told him to imagine that he had a rock resting on his right shoulder — a rock so heavy that it would prevent him from raising the shoulder. Ever since then this violinist has been walking around with a heavy (albeit imaginary) rock on his right shoulder.

The main fault with the rock image as a teaching device was that it replaced one poor habit of use with another. It would have been much more constructive to teach the student to eliminate the tension that caused the bad habit, rather than bury it under more tension.

Unfortunately, body problems are more the rule than the exception among performing artists. The Alexander Technique provides a solution to the practicing dilemma by eliminating the misuse that leads to such difficulties. Incorporated into early artistic training, the technique greatly reduces the likelihood of musculoskeletal problems developing. It is therefore included in the curriculum of many schools for the performing arts.

Donlin Foreman, principal dancer with the Martha Graham Company, would have avoided serious back trouble had he received better guidance regarding the use of his body as a beginning student. Don compressed his lower back so severely during his early years of training and performing that the nerve roots of the sciatic nerves became entrapped, causing weakness and pain in both legs. As Don puts it, "I took the physical pressure and emotional tension of dancing in my low back." He eventually had to have surgery to free the nerves. Following surgery, Don started using the Alexander Technique to "consciously allow my back to expand when I am dancing, instead of getting into a contracted state." He adds, "Surgeons can mechanically free the nerves, but if the way you work doesn't change, then you will have a relapse."

Learning a difficult skill, such as one of the performing arts, is often accompanied by mental and physical tensions that soon become habitual and keep the body from working efficiently. This occurs particularly when the learning is done in an environment that emphasizes achievement rather than efficient use of our psychophysical selves. As we use our conscious awareness to learn skilled activities, so, too, must we use it to detect and eliminate harmful habits that interfere with performing these skills efficiently.

A NEW WAY TO PRACTICE

Performing artists who have applied the Alexander Technique to their practicing have become aware of an interesting phenomenon: when their main focus is on their mind-body integration rather than on the specific demands of their art form, they are better able to fulfill their technical and artistic potential. Alexander described this way of working as concentrating on the "means whereby" rather than on the end result.

As you practice, I want you to interrupt yourself every time you become aware of unnecessary muscle tension or faulty postural habits. Interruptions can be frustrating, so please keep in mind the purpose, which is to identify and eliminate your faulty habits *within the context* of your practicing. You will have to change your priorities and consider the *process* of your practicing more important than the results.

This is how I want you to practice:

1. Select a piece of music, a dramatic scene, or a dance sequence you are currently working on.

2. Begin by saying no to your intention to practice. A deliberate decision to give up your intent to practice will prevent your old habits from instantly taking over, and allow a new way of using your body to take their place.

3. Silently instruct yourself in the Concepts of Good Use:

Allow your neck muscles to release so that your head can balance forward and up.
Allow your torso to release into length and width.
Allow your legs to release away from your pelvis.
Allow your shoulders to release out to the sides.

Repeat these four Concepts to yourself a few times, letting your body become quiet so that you can detect any muscular tensions that are contrary to them. You will feel your body respond by gradually becoming muscularly free and better aligned and balanced. You may also realize that you have more energy. This method of sending mental instructions to the different parts of your body is an excellent way of freeing and directing your energy so that it is more available for practicing and performing.

4. Start practicing. Stay aware of the four Concepts as you work—remember, they are your first priority. Use the Concepts as your guide to evaluate and correct your use.

5. Stop practicing as soon as you become aware of falling into your old habits of misuse. Each time you stop, say no again to the idea of practicing, then focus on the four Concepts before resuming.

The most important aspect of working in this way is to keep your thoughts focused on your head-neck-torso integration. Gradually your improved use will last for longer periods and will begin to carry over into your performances.

PRACTICAL BENEFITS

Alexander's Concepts are helpful for achieving an awareness of the body as a whole, which is extremely important for all performing artists. The body that is the vehicle for your artistic self can become a jumble of functionally disorganized parts unless you have a way of conceptually organizing your entire self. If you are a pianist, for example, your fingers can have the power and dexterity to follow the music you hear inside you only when your wrists and arms are free, and they can be free only when your shoulders are correctly balanced. Balanced shoulders can occur only when your torso is lengthening and widening, which in turn requires your head to be correctly balanced and your hip joints released. Good head-neck-torso integration enables your fingers to receive power from the large back muscles and remain free enough to do their skilled work.

FOR DANCERS: PERFORMING WITH AN INJURY

Were logic the only governing force in our lives, no one would dance with an injury. However, due to necessity in some cases and inner needs in others, dancers with injuries are frequently found in class, at rehearsal, and on stage. Performing with an injury can lead to further injury if not done with care.

You can prevent the damaging compensation that often follows injury by using Alexander's Concepts of Good Use to guide your body. You will also help correct the tension and malalignment that may have precipitated the injury in the first place. You should not let your need to protect an injured part of the body—such as being careful the knee bends over the foot or you turn out from the hip joints—cause you to focus only on that injured part. Your need to protect the injury should be integrated into an awareness of the body as a whole. An excellent way of doing this is to think of the head leading the spine into length while at the same time being aware of the specific part of the body that needs protecting.

DEALING WITH EMOTIONAL DYNAMICS

Actors who want to portray emotional conflict coupled with mounting body tension must move the audience to feel what they are feeling, but they must not hurt themselves in the process. Some performers, in a desire to reach the audience, turn their energy into damaging body tension. Actors, for example, have been known to develop nodes on their vocal cords after holding tension in the throat. Actors, musicians, and dancers must all learn to express emotional and dynamic intensity without "locking up" their energy.

You may be able to solve this problem with an approach that worked for me when I was performing as a modern dancer. I would use Alexander's four Concepts to create a visual image of my entire body, and then visualize my energy flowing freely through this image. Because the Concepts consist of releasing muscles and directing energy throughout the body, they prevented me from becoming held or locked in one local area.

ADDITIONAL BENEFITS

Alexander's work can do much more than help overcome painful body problems for the performer. It can bring the performer's body under more conscious control and therefore increase its versatility as an instrument for artistic expression.

Conductors can get better results from their orchestras because they are more in touch with the way they use the energy in their bodies. Actors can eliminate unwanted idiosyncratic gestures and postures they might otherwise bring to the characterizations they portray.

I have heard some performers say that the Alexander Technique has helped them deal with stage fright. By taking time to review the Concepts of Good Use just before going on stage, they achieve a mind-body centering that prevents performance anxiety.

Having emphasized the importance of keeping your thoughts focused on your head-neck-torso integration as you practice, rather than on the results, I thought you might be interested in reading Alexander's own words on this most important point:

> *For if the pupil thinks of a certain "end" as desirable and starts to pursue it directly, he will certainly take the course of action that he has been accustomed to take in like conditions. In other words, he will follow his habitual procedure in regard to it, and should that procedure happen to be a bad one for the purpose, he only strengthens the incorrect experiences in connection with it by using this procedure again. If, on the other hand, the pupil* stops himself *from going to work in his usual way (inhibition), and proceeds to replace his old subconscious means by the new conscious means which his teacher has given him, he will have taken the first and most important step towards the breaking-down of a habit, and towards that constructive, conscious and reasoning control which tends towards a mastery of the situation. It is therefore impressed on the pupil from the beginning that, as the essential preliminary to any successful work on his part,* he must refuse to work directly for his "end," *and keep his attention on the means whereby this end can be achieved.*

(from *Constructive Conscious Control of the Individual*)

15

Pregnancy and Back Pain

BACK PAIN IS NOT unusual during pregnancy. For most women the pain goes away after the baby is born, but for a large minority it remains, developing into chronic back trouble.

As the body prepares for birth, normal hormonal changes cause the ligaments of the spine and pelvis to become more elastic so that they give less support. This factor, plus the weight of the baby, increases the harmful effects of poor postural habits and sets the stage for back problems.

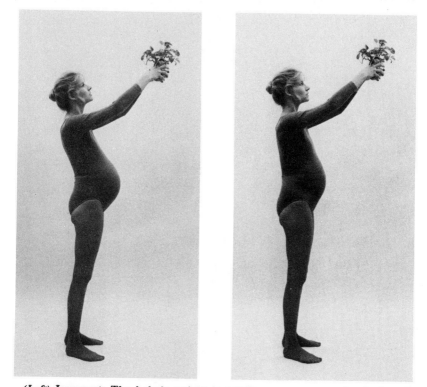

(Left) **Incorrect: The baby's weight is causing more compression in Janet's lower back than necessary.** *(Right)* **Correct: The baby's weight is more efficiently dealt with as Janet's head leads her spine into length, and her torso lengthens and widens. Janet's entire body is better balanced.**

The effectiveness of improved muscular support in reducing the postural stresses of pregnancy is evident in the accompanying photographs of Janet, taken two weeks before her baby was born. Compare the alignment of Janet's head, neck, and torso in the two pictures. In the left-hand picture, her head is pulled back and down and the weight of the baby is causing her back to become arched and compressed. In the right-hand picture, her head is releasing forward and up, and she is dealing with the baby's weight more effectively by lengthening and widening her back.

Keeping width in your back is particularly important during pregnancy. As the baby grows and gives your body more weight in front, it becomes even more important to keep your lower back wide instead of arching it, to counterbalance the weight. Sitting

with a lengthened spine will also enable your back to deal with
the weight of the baby more efficiently.

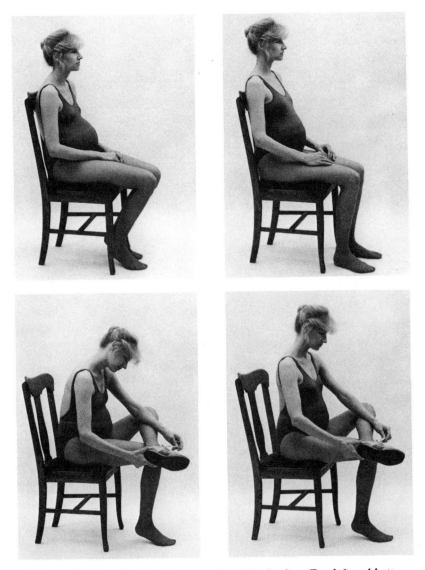

Sitting with the spine lengthened protects the back. *(Top left and bottom left)* **Incorrect.** *(Top right and bottom right)* **Correct.**

A dramatic difference in neck and upper back alignment is illustrated in the pictures below, which show incorrect and correct bending. As you look at the photo of Janet bending correctly, notice the length in her neck and back. She is allowing her head to lead her spine into length and her torso to lengthen and widen. You should do the same as you practice bending.

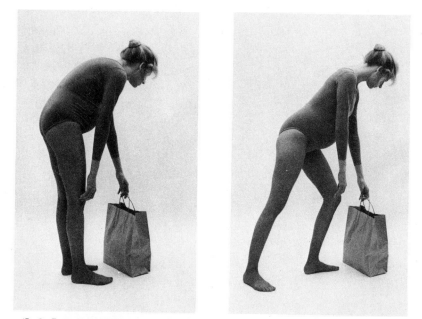

(Left) Incorrect. *(Right)* **Correct: Notice the dramatic difference in neck and upper back alignment. The incorrect use is harmful to the back and neck as well as being less attractive.**

There is no denying that your abdominal muscles become stretched during pregnancy, but they need not become weak. Exercising your abdominal muscles while lying down is valuable, but it will not train them to work for you while you are up and moving around. I recommend, therefore, that throughout your pregnancy you supplement your lying-down exercises by briefly tightening your lower abdominals five times every two hours as you go about your daily activities. You can check to see if you are doing the exercise correctly by placing your hand just below your belly button to feel the muscles contract. Your abdominal muscles will also be encouraged to work every time you remind yourself to widen, rather than arch, your back. Keeping your abdominal muscles strong will help you stay in shape during pregnancy and get your figure back quickly after the baby is born.

Janet has this to say about the importance of good use during pregnancy: "I found that everything I did was more difficult. Every bad postural habit I had became exaggerated and caused more pressure on my body. I became much more conscious of needing length and width in my back when I was far along in my pregnancy."

For Janet, the biggest obstacle to good use, once her baby was born, was her tendency to round her upper back by "going down to the baby," as she put it. She says, "You should think of bringing the baby up to you." Raise the height of the changing table, if necessary.

When nursing the baby, be sure to use a chair that gives good back support. If the chair does not support your arms, place pillows under your elbows. And, most important, use a large enough pillow under the baby to raise him or her up so you do not have to slump.

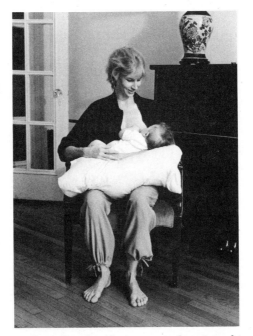

Position your baby as Janet has done here, so you do not need to slump down while nursing.

Conclusion

YOU ARE THE POSSESSOR of one of Nature's most elegant inventions—the human spine, with all its surrounding structures. Your *back*, as this entire possession is called, is extremely versatile and capable. Back pain is not part of your evolutionary heritage; it need not be the price you pay for the luxury of walking on two feet.

I realize that the solution I have offered for your back pain is not as simple as taking a pill or being the recipient of passive forms of treatment. But the nature of back pain precludes these easy answers. I am confident, however, that applying what you have learned will be an enjoyable as well as healing experience.

Your body goes everywhere you go, and so does your mind. Having both exist in harmony, beneficially interacting, can add a great deal to your daily enjoyment of life and your sense of well-being.

Sources of Information on the Alexander Technique

FURTHER READING

If the following titles are not available locally, many of them can be ordered from: Centerline Press, 2005 Palo Verde Ave., Suite 325, Long Beach, California 90815.

Alexander, F. M., *The Use of the Self*, Centerline Press, 1985.

Barker, S., *The Alexander Technique: The Revolutionary Way to Use Your Body for Total Energy*, Bantam Books, New York, 1978.

Barlow, W., *The Alexander Technique*, Warner Books, New York, 1980.

Gelb, M., *Body Learning: An Introduction to the Alexander Technique*, Aurum Press, London, 1981.

Jones, F. P., *Body Awareness in Action: A Study of the Alexander Technique*, Schocken Books, New York, 1979.

Maisel, E., ed., *The Resurrection of the Body--The Essential Writings of F.M. Alexander*, Shambhala Inc., Boston, 1986.

Stransky, J. with Stone, R., *The Alexander Technique: Joy in the Life of Your Body*, Beaufort Books, New York, 1981.

FOR GENERAL INFORMATION

The American Center for the Alexander Technique, Inc.
129 West 67th Street
New York, NY 10023
(212) 799-0468

The North American Society of Teachers of the Alexander Technique,
   Inc.
P. O. Box 806
Ansonia Station
New York, NY 10023
(212) 866-5640

The Society of Teachers of the Alexander Technique
10 London House
266 Fulham Road
London SW10 9EL
England

Index

T